Vishal Saini M.D. FAASM

BEYOND CPAP
NEW HOPE FOR SLEEP APNEA

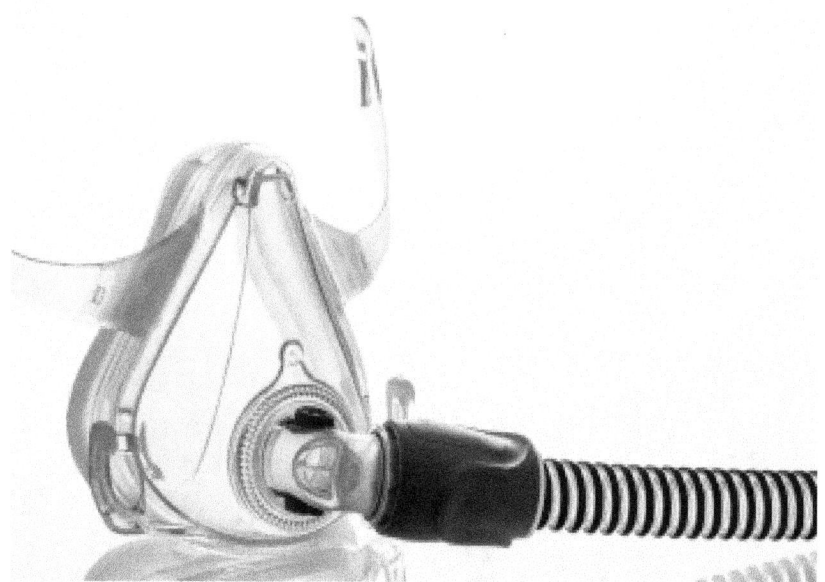

BEYOND

CPAP

NEW HOPE FOR

SLEEP APNEA

By

Vishal Saini M.D. FAASM

Copyright © 2025 by Vishal Saini M.D. FAASM

All rights reserved. No part of this publication may be reproduced, stored in a retrieval system, or transmitted in any form or by any means, electronic, mechanical, photocopying, recording, or otherwise, without the prior written permission of the publisher

Contents

About the Author 1

Foreword 3

Chapter 1 A Wake-Up Call 5

You're Not Just Tired—Something is Stealing Your Sleep 5

What's Inside 6

Definition of Sleep Apnea 7

Obstructive Sleep Apnea (OSA) 8

Self-Assessment: Check Your Airway with the Mallampati Score 9

How to Check: 9

Interpreting Your Score: 10

What Happens During an OSA Episode 11

Central Sleep Apnea (CSA) 12

The Brain's Breathing Control Center 12

Neurological Triggers of Central Sleep Apnea 13

How CSA Differs from OSA 14

Complex Sleep Apnea Syndrome 16

The Puzzling Emergence 17

Did you know? 17

Why Does CPAP Trigger Central Apneas? 17

Identifying Complex Sleep Apnea 18

Prevalence and Demographics 19

The Geographic Picture 19

The Gender Gap 20

The Age Factor 22

Identifying Symptoms 24

Nighttime Warning Signs 24

How Symptoms Differ By Type 26

Diagnosis through Sleep Studies 28

The Berlin Questionnaire: A Time-Tested Tool 29

STOP-BANG: The Gold Standard for Surgical Patients 30

The Multi-Level Approach to Risk Assessment 30

Key Categories in Sleep Apnea Stratification 31

Severity-Based Categories 31

Treatment History Categories 31

Anatomical Categories 32

Choosing a Testing Method 32

In-Lab Polysomnography: The Gold Standard 33

Limitations of In-Lab Sleep Studies 34

Cardiovascular Risk and Complications 35

Hypertension: The Silent Connection 36

Heart Disease and Stroke Risk 37

Neurological and Cognitive Effects.. 38

The Oxygen Deprivation Cascade 38

Everyday Cognitive Challenges 39

Emotional and Psychological Impact 41

Metabolic and Hormonal Impact 42

The Insulin Resistance Connection 42

Hunger Hormones Gone Haywire 43

The Metabolic Syndrome Connection 44

Endurance under Siege 46

Reaction Time and Decision-Making.. 47

CPAP Therapy Overview 48

How CPAP Works: A Gentle Air Splint 49

The Components of a CPAP System 49

Effectiveness: The Numbers Tell the Story 50

Challenges and Compliance Issues... 51

Physical Discomfort and Mask Issues 51

Psychological and Emotional Barriers.. 52

Conclusion and Transition 53

Chapter 2: The Science behind Sleep Implants 56

Historical Development of Sleep Implants..................................... 56

Inspire™ Upper Airway Stimulation 59

Types of Sleep Implants 60

Hypoglossal Nerve Stimulation (HNS) Implants 60

Phrenic Nerve Stimulation Systems 61

Emerging Implant Technologies 62

Technical Anatomy of Sleep Implants 62

The Pulse Generator: The Brain of the Operation 63

The Breathing Sensor: Your Sleep's Vigilant Guardian 63

The Stimulation Lead: The Vital Connection 64

Design Considerations in Sleep Implants 65

Biocompatibility: Making Friends with the Body 65

Power Efficiency: The Battery Life Challenge 66

Size and Ergonomics: The Comfort Factor 66

Efficacy Studies: Sleep Implants vs. CPAP 67

The Numbers Game: AHI Reduction 67

Beyond Numbers: Quality of Life Improvements 69

Quality of Life Improvements with Sleep Implants 69

Safety Profiles of Sleep Implants 71

Understanding the Risks: Surgical Considerations 71

Long-Term Safety: What the Data Shows 73

Surgical and Post-Surgical Considerations 74

The Surgical Journey 74

Immediate Post-Operative Care.. 75

The Healing Phase 75

Next-Generation Sleep Implants... 77

Smart Polymer Implants: The Flexible Future 77

Miniaturized and Battery-Free Designs.................................... 78

Artificial Intelligence and Adaptive Stimulation...................... 79

Conclusion and Transition... 80

Chapter 3: Types of Sleep Implants and Their Application 82

Exploring the Implant Landscape.. 82

Patient Eligibility for HNS 83

Looking Inside: The Critical Airway Assessment..................... 85

What Happens During a DISE Procedure?............................... 86

Key Observations in DISE.. 86

Why DISE Matters for HNS Success 87

Clinical Evidence of HNS 87

Comparing Apples to Apples: HNS vs. CPAP.......................... 88

Future Directions in HNS Technology 89

Role of Dental Implants in OSA.. 89

Combination Therapy Options 92

CPAP and Implant Therapy: Unexpected Partners 92

Positional Therapy: A Simple but Powerful Addition 93

Exercise: Beyond Just Weight Loss 94

Targeted Upper Airway Exercises 95

Sleep Positioning and Bedroom Environment 96

Conclusion and Transition 98

Chapter 4: The Patient Journey with Sleep Implants 100

The Road to Restorative Sleep 100

Patient Testimonials: Overcoming Initial Challenges 101

The First Few Days: Surgical Recovery Hurdles 102

The Waiting Game: Activation Anticipation 103

Finding the Sweet Spot: Titration Challenges 104

Narrative: Life after Sleep Implants 104

The Transformation Timeline 104

Sleep Quality: The Foundation of Everything 106

Daytime Energy: Reclaiming Waking Hours 106

Integrating Sleep Implants into Daily Life 107

The Nightly Ritual: Activating Your Silent Partner 107

Adjusting to the Sensations 108

Fine-Tuning for Comfort and Effectiveness 110

Optimizing Health and Well-Being Post-Implants 110

Beyond the Device: Creating a Holistic Recovery Plan 111

Nutrition: Fueling Your Recovery and Beyond 111

Movement: Finding Your Exercise Sweet Spot 112

Conclusion and Transition 113

Chapter 5: Metabolic Enhancement and Integrating GLP1 Therapies with Sleep Implants 116

Exploring Metabolic Dysregulation in Sleep Apnea 116

The Obesity Connection: More than Just Weight 117

Impact of Weight Loss on Sleep Apnea and Implants 118

How Weight Loss Enhances Sleep Implant Effectiveness 119

Sustainable Weight Loss Strategies for Sleep Apnea Patients .. 120

Definition and Mechanism of GLP-1 Receptor Agonists........... 122

How GLP-1 Agonists Work: A Multi-System Approach.......... 123

Brain Effects: Appetite Control 123

Digestive System: Slowing Things Down 124

Introduction to Zepbound as an Adjunct Therapy 124

Zepbound and Sleep Implants: A Powerful Combination 125

Beyond Weight Loss: Metabolic Benefits for Sleep Apnea 125

Effectiveness and Mechanics of Zepbound 126

How Zepbound Transforms Breathing during Sleep 127

Review of Clinical Studies on GLP-1 in Sleep Apnea 128

Beyond Zepbound: The Broader GLP-1 Evidence Base 129

Mechanisms beyond Weight Loss 129

GLP-1 and Implant Therapy 130

Measurable Improvements in Sleep Parameters 131

Quality of Life Transformations 132

Developing Integrative Treatment Protocols 133

Step-by-Step Protocol Development... 133

Comprehensive Initial Assessment 134

Establish Treatment Sequence 134

Implement Continuous Monitoring... 134

Coordinate Supportive Care... 135

Patient Selection and Treatment Personalization...................... 135

Personalization Factors That Enhance Success 136

Sleep Apnea Phenotype 136

Metabolic Health Assessment.. 137

Side Effect Management... 137

Cost and Access Barriers 137

Coordination of Care Challenges.. 138

Gradual Dose Adjustments and Dietary Modifications 139

Maximizing Insurance Coverage and Financial Assistance 139

Personalized Therapy Adjustments... 140

Long-Term Monitoring and Lifestyle Integration 140

Conclusion and Transition 141

Chapter 6: Innovations and Future Directions 144

Reimagining Sleep Apnea Treatment 144

Neurostimulation Devices 145

How Neurostimulation Works 145

The Inspire System: Leading the Revolution 146

AI-Driven Therapy Customization 147

Real-Time Adaptation 147

Learning From Your Sleep Patterns 148

Personalized Therapy without Doctor Visits 149

Miniaturization and Design Innovations 149

The Shrinking Footprint 149

Material Innovations Driving Change 150

Power Efficiency: Doing More with Less 151

Introduction to Personalized Medicine 151

Role of AI in Personalized Treatment 152

Dynamic Treatment Adjustment 153

Genetic Data and Treatment Optimization 154

Matching Genetics to Treatment Options 155

Predicting Treatment Response 155

Overview of Market Growth and Opportunities 156

Current Market Landscape 156

Growth Projections and Opportunities 157

Regional Market Expansion 158

Technological Innovations and Next-Generation Implants 158

Expanding Patient Eligibility and Awareness 159

Regulatory Challenges in Implant Approval 160

Post-Approval Monitoring and Risk Management 161

Effective Educational Strategies 163

Multi-Modal Learning 163

Peer Support Programs 163

Conclusion 164

About the Author

Dr. Vishal Saini, M.D., FAASM

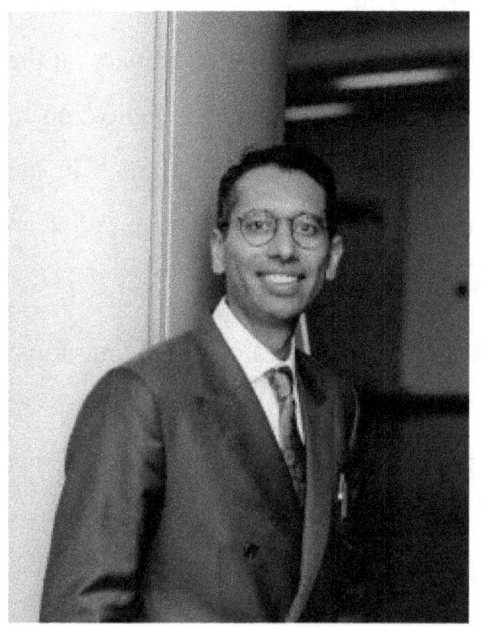

What if the key to unlocking better sleep wasn't just about forcing air through a mask but about working with the body's own mechanisms? That question has driven Dr. Vishal Saini to the forefront of sleep medicine innovation.

Dr. Saini isn't just a physician—he's a problem solver, a researcher, and a relentless advocate for patients struggling with sleep disorders. As the research and medical director at the Midwest Center for Sleep Disorders, he has spent his career exploring new frontiers in sleep medicine, particularly for patients who can't tolerate traditional treatments like CPAP.

His work is more than just clinical—under his leadership, sleep labs have expanded access to care, introduced cutting-edge research trials, and explored groundbreaking alternatives for patients with rare and complex sleep disorders. His contributions don't stop in the lab or clinic; as an assistant clinical professor at Michigan State University and President of the Michigan Academy of Sleep Medicine, he's shaping the future of sleep medicine for the next generation.

In recognition of his contributions, Dr. Saini was named a Fellow of the American Academy of Sleep Medicine (FAASM) in 2025, a distinction awarded to leaders who have made a lasting impact on the field through research, education, and patient care. His dedication to advancing sleep medicine has positioned him as a key voice in the evolution of treatment options, particularly in the development of sleep implants and other innovative therapies.

At the heart of Dr. Saini's work is a belief that sleep medicine must evolve. His research into alternative treatments and personalized solutions is paving the way for new possibilities. This book, like his career, is about going beyond the status quo—because for millions struggling with sleep apnea, better solutions aren't just nice to have. They're necessary.

Foreword

This book is dedicated to all my patients who I have served over the years in their health journeys. I first learned about hypoglossal nerve implant therapy trials, which were finishing up in 2013-2014, when I was still doing my sleep medicine fellowship at Wayne State University in Detroit, MI. In 2021, I introduced Inspire therapy for the first time in our Mid-Michigan Tri-City area clinic due to burgeoning demand from sleep apnea patients seeking alternative treatment options. Over the last four years, hundreds of patients have been able to use these newer therapies and achieve better sleep.

I am writing this book to capture essential information that a reader, whether it's a patient who is considering alternative options, a spouse who wants better sleep for their partner and for themselves, or whether you are a healthcare provider looking out for your patient's best interest; will find very useful and explain not just the science of sleep apnea treatments but also practical considerations when you are approaching these novel therapies.

This work would not be possible without inspiration and love from my wife, Shivani, and my children, Neil and Claire. I thank them all for putting up with the demands on my time.

Wish you a better sleep ahead. Tathastu!

Vishal Saini, MD, FAASM Lansing, MI

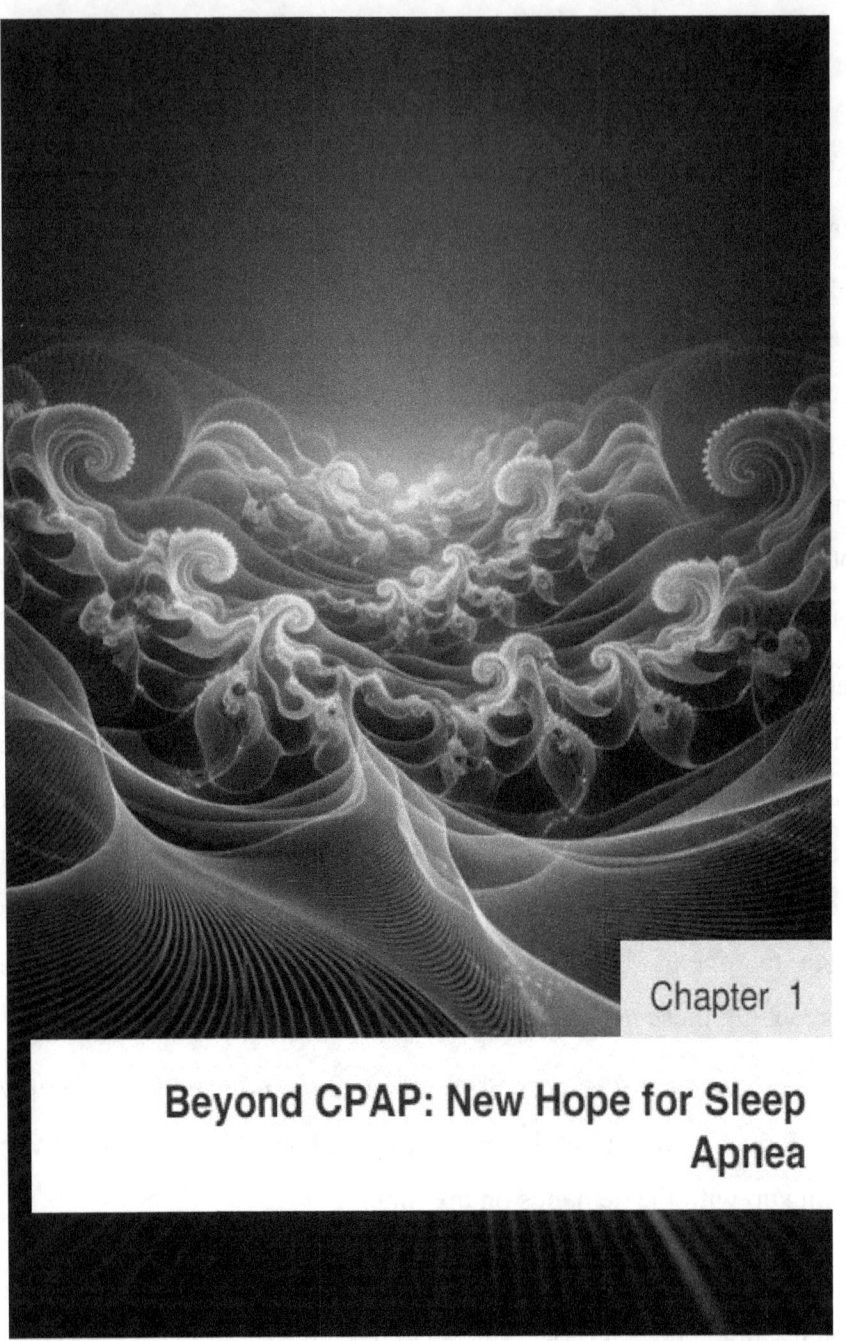

Chapter 1

Beyond CPAP: New Hope for Sleep Apnea

Chapter 1 A Wake-Up Call

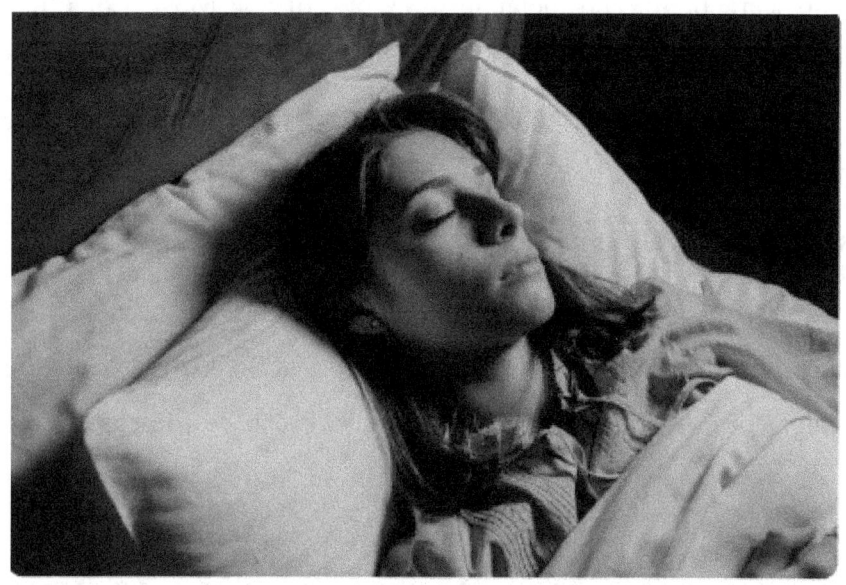

Photo credit: Pexels.

You're Not Just Tired—Something is Stealing Your Sleep

Ever wake up feeling like you've been hit by a truck, even though you got a full night's sleep? Or maybe your partner nudges you in the middle of the night, complaining that you sound like a chainsaw in overdrive? What if I told you that, while you're peacefully snoozing, your body might be gasping for air—sometimes hundreds of times per night—without you even knowing it?

Welcome to the sneaky, silent world of sleep apnea, a condition that turns every night into an invisible battle for oxygen.

For years, sleep apnea has been a frustrating puzzle for millions. It zaps your energy, messes with your mood, and can even wreak havoc on your heart, brain, and metabolism. Worst of all? Most people don't even realize they have it until years—or even decades—have passed. The symptoms hide in plain sight, dismissed as just "getting older" or "normal tiredness."

But what if there was a better way to fight back?

For a long time, the go-to treatment for sleep apnea has been the CPAP machine—that bulky, air-blasting mask that looks like something straight out of a sci-fi movie. While CPAP can be life-changing for some, let's be real: many people find it uncomfortable, inconvenient, or downright impossible to use. So what happens if CPAP isn't for you? Are you doomed to a lifetime of exhaustion, brain fog, and increased health risks?

Absolutely not.

This book is your guide to the new frontier of sleep apnea treatment—one that goes beyond CPAP. We're talking about sleep implants—tiny, high-tech devices that work inside your body to restore natural breathing and give you back the deep, uninterrupted sleep you deserve.

What's Inside

We'll start by breaking down what sleep apnea actually is—what causes it, how it messes with your body, and why traditional treatments don't always work for everyone. Then, we'll dive into the game-changing world of sleep implants—how they work, who they're for, and what the latest research says about their effectiveness.

But we won't stop there. This book isn't just about technology—it's about giving you the power to take control of your sleep health. From understanding the latest innovations to navigating treatment options, insurance, and real-world success stories, you'll come away with the knowledge you need to make the best decisions for your health.

By the end of this journey, you won't just be another sleep apnea statistic. You'll be informed, empowered, and ready to reclaim your nights—and your life. So take a deep breath (while you're awake, at least), and let's dive in. The future of sleep apnea treatment is here, and it's time to wake up to the possibilities.

Definition of Sleep Apnea

When people think of sleep disorders, insomnia often comes to mind first. But imagine something potentially more serious happening while you sleep—your breathing repeatedly stops and starts throughout the night, sometimes hundreds of times, without you even knowing it. This is sleep apnea, a common but frequently undiagnosed condition affecting millions worldwide.

At its core, sleep apnea is a breathing disorder that occurs during sleep. The word "apnea" comes from Greek, meaning "without breath," and that's precisely what happens—breathing pauses or becomes very shallow during sleep. These pauses can last from a few seconds to minutes and may occur 30 or more times per hour in severe cases. Sleep apnea can happen in two main ways. The most common type, obstructive sleep apnea (OSA), occurs when the airway becomes blocked, restricting airflow to the lungs. The second type, central sleep apnea (CSA), happens when the brain fails to send the proper signals to the muscles that control breathing, causing pauses or shallow breaths.

Obstructive Sleep Apnea (OSA)

Imagine trying to breathe through a straw that keeps getting pinched shut. That's essentially what happens with obstructive sleep apnea (OSA), the most common form of sleep apnea affecting millions worldwide. While you sleep peacefully, a silent battle takes place in your airway dozens or even hundreds of times each night.

OSA occurs when the muscles supporting your upper airway relax too much during sleep. This relaxation isn't the pleasant kind that helps you drift off to dreamland—it's a mechanical problem that can have serious health consequences. When these muscles relax excessively, the airway narrows or closes completely as you try to breathe in, temporarily cutting off your oxygen supply.

Understanding Obstructive Sleep Apnea (OSA)

Understanding what physically happens during an OSA episode helps explain why some people are more vulnerable than others. Your upper airway is essentially a tube of soft tissue that can collapse inward when muscle tone decreases during sleep. Several key structures play a role in this collapse:

- The soft palate (the soft tissue at the back of the roof of your mouth) can sag downward.
- Your tongue, which is actually a large muscle, can relax and fall backward.
- The uvula (that dangling tissue at the back of your throat) and tonsils can further narrow the already compromised space.
- In some people, even the lateral walls of the throat contribute to the obstruction by collapsing inward.

Think of your airway like a garden hose—when it's fully open, air flows freely. But any pinching or pressure can restrict or completely block that flow. Unlike a garden hose, though, your airway is made of soft, collapsible tissue that needs muscle activity to stay open.

Self-Assessment: Check Your Airway with the Mallampati Score

One way to assess your risk for obstructive sleep apnea is by evaluating your Mallampati Score, which measures how much of your airway is visible when you open your mouth.

How to Check:

- Stand in front of a mirror.
- Open your mouth wide and stick your tongue out without saying "Ahhh" or making any sound.
- Compare what you see with the images below.

Interpreting Your Score:

- Class 1 & 2: More of the airway is visible, meaning a lower risk of obstruction.
- Class 3 & 4: Less of the airway is visible, indicating a narrow airway, which is a risk factor for obstructive sleep apnea.

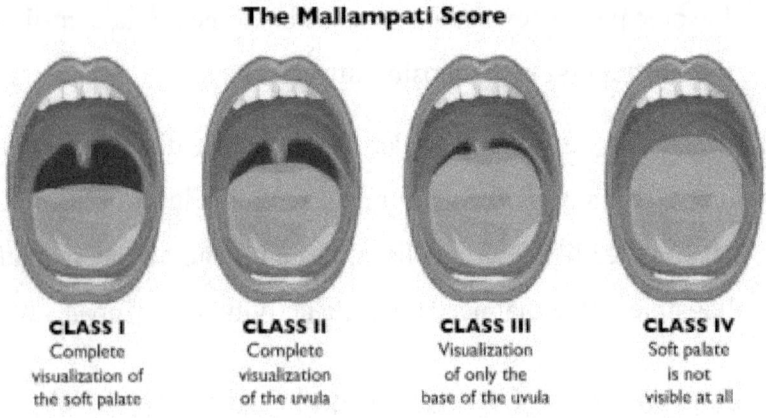

Illustration: Mallampati Score Chart, Clinical Advisor (2016)

If your score is Class 3 or 4, you may have a higher risk for sleep apnea and should consider discussing it with a healthcare professional.

Did you know?

The narrowest part of your airway is behind your tongue and soft palate. This region, called the velopharynx, is where most obstructions occur in OSA. Imaging studies have shown that the velopharynx is significantly smaller in people with OSA compared to those without the condition, even when awake. Research published in the *Journal of Applied Physiology* found that the cross-sectional area of the velopharynx can decrease by up to 66% during inspiratory flow limitation, highlighting how anatomical and functional differences contribute to airway collapse during sleep.

What Happens During an OSA Episode

An OSA episode follows a distinct pattern:

- First, as you drift into sleep, your airway muscles begin to relax. For most people, this relaxation is moderate and doesn't cause problems. However, in those with OSA, the relaxation becomes excessive, narrowing the airway significantly.
- As you inhale, the negative pressure created by your breathing efforts actually pulls the relaxed tissues together, further blocking the airway—like trying to suck through a straw that's collapsing. You continue making breathing efforts, with your chest and diaphragm moving, but little or no air gets through.
- Oxygen levels in your blood begin to drop while carbon dioxide levels rise. Your brain, sensing this dangerous situation, triggers what sleep specialists call an "arousal response"—a protective mechanism that briefly wakes you just enough to tighten those airway muscles and open the passage.

This arousal is typically accompanied by a gasp, snort, or body jerk as you suddenly resume breathing. While you rarely fully awaken or remember these episodes, they disrupt your sleep cycle and prevent you from reaching or maintaining the deeper, restorative stages of sleep.

Then, as you settle back into sleep, the cycle begins again—sometimes repeating dozens of times per hour in severe cases. Each episode is like a mini-emergency for your body, triggering stress hormones and placing strain on your cardiovascular system.

Central Sleep Apnea (CSA)

While obstructive sleep apnea happens when your airway gets blocked, central sleep apnea (CSA) is a different story altogether. With CSA, the airway remains open, but your brain temporarily stops sending the signals that tell your body to breathe. It's as if the respiratory control center in your brain takes an unscheduled break, leaving your breathing muscles without instructions.

> This neurological glitch creates a dangerous situation your body literally forgets to breathe for brief periods during sleep. Unlike the gasping or choking that often accompanies OSA, people with pure central sleep apnea may have quieter episodes, making the condition even more difficult to detect without proper testing.

The Brain's Breathing Control Center

To understand central sleep apnea, we need to appreciate how breathing normally works during sleep. Your brainstem, specifically areas called the medulla and pons, contains your respiratory control center. This remarkable system automatically adjusts your breathing rate and depth based on the levels of oxygen and carbon dioxide in your blood.

During wakefulness, you have both automatic breathing control and voluntary control (like when you hold your breath). During sleep, however, breathing becomes entirely dependent on this automatic system. If something interferes with these brain signals, breathing can temporarily stop, creating a central apnea event.

Did you know?

Your body's response to carbon dioxide (CO_2) levels plays a more crucial role in breathing regulation than oxygen levels. Even small increases in CO_2 normally trigger the brain to increase breathing, as central chemoreceptors in the medulla detect these changes and stimulate ventilation. Research published in the American Journal of Respiratory and Critical Care Medicine found that in some forms of central sleep apnea (CSA), particularly in heart failure patients, this CO_2 sensitivity becomes heightened, leading to unstable breathing patterns and periodic apneas.

During a central apnea episode, unlike obstructive apnea, there's no struggle to breathe against a blocked airway. Instead, the chest and abdomen remain still because the brain isn't activating the respiratory muscles. After several seconds (sometimes up to a minute or more), the brain's monitoring system detects the rising carbon dioxide or falling oxygen and "reboots" the breathing signal, often causing the person to wake briefly as breathing resumes.

Neurological Triggers of Central Sleep Apnea

Several neurological conditions and factors can disrupt the brain's breathing control system:

- Brainstem damage: Strokes, tumors, infections, or injuries affecting the brainstem can damage the respiratory control centers. Even a seemingly unrelated stroke in other parts of the brain can sometimes affect pathways that influence breathing regulation.

- Neurodegenerative diseases: Conditions like Parkinson's disease, multiple system atrophy, and other disorders that affect the nervous system can disrupt the neural pathways involved in breathing control.
- Spinal cord injuries: Damage to the upper spinal cord, especially the cervical region, can interrupt the nerve signals between the brain and the breathing muscles.
- Medication effects: Opioid medications (like morphine, oxycodone, and fentanyl) are powerful respiratory depressants that can cause central sleep apnea even in people with no previous sleep issues. These medications reduce the brain's sensitivity to carbon dioxide, dampening the drive to breathe.

Heart failure also commonly causes a specific form of central sleep apnea called Cheyne-Stokes respiration. In this pattern, breathing gradually increases in depth, then decreases until breathing stops briefly before the cycle repeats. This happens because heart failure creates a delay in the feedback loop between the lungs and brain due to slowed blood circulation.

How CSA Differs from OSA

While both obstructive sleep apnea (OSA) and central sleep apnea (CSA) lead to breathing pauses during sleep, they are driven by very different mechanisms. OSA involves a physical blockage in the airway, whereas CSA is the result of a communication failure between the brain and the breathing muscles. Here's how the two conditions differ across key aspects:

- Cause of Apnea:

OSA is caused by a physical collapse or blockage of the upper airway.

CSA occurs when the brain temporarily fails to send the signal to breathe.

- Breathing Effort:

In OSA, the chest and diaphragm continue making efforts to breathe despite the blocked airway.

In CSA, there is no breathing effort at all during the pause.

- Typical Symptoms:

OSA often involves loud snoring, gasping, or choking sounds.

CSA episodes are usually quieter and may go unnoticed without a sleep study.

- Diagnostic Clues:

OSA can sometimes be suspected based on physical traits (like a high Mallampati Score).

CSA requires specialized testing to observe brain-controlled breathing patterns.

- Who It Affects:

OSA is more common in people who are overweight, have narrow airways, or have sleep-related muscle relaxation issues.

CSA often affects individuals with heart failure, neurological disorders, or those using opioid medications.

Understanding these differences is crucial for accurate diagnosis and treatment. Central sleep apnea requires a focus on neurological factors, while obstructive sleep apnea often involves physical interventions to keep the airway open.

Complex Sleep Apnea Syndrome

Imagine this scenario: After struggling with loud snoring and daytime sleepiness for years, Michael finally undergoes a sleep study and is diagnosed with obstructive sleep apnea. He receives a CPAP machine, excited to finally get a good night's sleep. But something unexpected happens while the machine successfully opens his airway; he now experiences new breathing pauses where he simply stops breathing altogether despite the open airway. Michael has developed what sleep specialists call complex sleep apnea syndrome.

Complex sleep apnea syndrome (CompSAS), also known as treatment-emergent central sleep apnea, represents a fascinating hybrid of sleep-disordered breathing. It occurs when someone who primarily has obstructive sleep apnea develops central sleep apneas during treatment with CPAP therapy. In other words, fixing one breathing problem unmasks or creates another.

The Puzzling Emergence

Studies, including those by Morgenthaler et al. in 2006 and Endo et al. in 2008, have found that 5–15% of patients undergoing CPAP treatment for obstructive sleep apnea begin experiencing central apneas that were not previously prominent. This phenomenon, known as treatment-emergent central apnea, may be temporary and often resolves with continued therapy.

During these central events, the airway remains open (thanks to the CPAP), but breathing stops because the brain temporarily fails to send signals to the respiratory muscles. This creates a frustrating situation the very treatment meant to solve breathing problems seems to create new ones.

Did you know?

Sleep specialists often define complex sleep apnea as the persistence or emergence of central apneas (5 or more per hour) during CPAP titration when the obstructive events have been eliminated. Some patients may have a mix of both central and obstructive events from the beginning, but the central component becomes more apparent once CPAP addresses the obstructive component.

Why Does CPAP Trigger Central Apneas?

The emergence of central apneas during CPAP therapy isn't fully understood, but several mechanisms likely contribute:

- Ventilatory control instability: Some people have a respiratory control system that overreacts to small changes in carbon dioxide levels, a phenomenon sleep specialists call "high loop gain." CPAP can make breathing more efficient, which might lower carbon dioxide levels enough to temporarily halt the brain's breathing signals.
- Pressure-induced changes: The positive pressure from CPAP might activate certain receptors in the lungs that affect breathing control. This is similar to how taking a very deep breath can momentarily make you pause before your next breath.
- Unmasking existing central tendencies: Some researchers believe complex sleep apnea patients may have had an underlying tendency toward central apneas all along, but these were "hidden" by the more obvious obstructive events. Once CPAP resolves the obstructions, the central breathing issues become apparent.

For many patients, these central events are most prominent when they first start CPAP therapy. The brain and body are essentially adjusting to a new breathing environment created by the machine.

Identifying Complex Sleep Apnea

Complex sleep apnea is typically identified during a sleep study when a patient is being fitted for a CPAP machine. As the technician adjusts the pressure to eliminate obstructive events, they may notice the emergence of central apneas on the monitoring equipment.

Some people with complex sleep apnea report feeling like they're "fighting" their CPAP machine or experiencing a sensation of being unable to exhale against the pressure. Others may feel like they're "forgetting to breathe" while using the device. These subjective experiences can provide clues, but proper diagnosis requires objective measurement in a sleep lab.

Prevalence and Demographics

Sleep apnea affects a staggering portion of the global population, though the numbers vary significantly depending on how we define and measure it. A 2019 study published in *The Lancet Respiratory Medicine* estimated that nearly one billion adults worldwide—yes, billion with a "b"—may have at least mild sleep apnea. Of these, approximately 425 million are believed to have moderate to severe cases that would likely benefit from treatment. This research, led by Benjafield and colleagues, analyzed global prevalence using standardized diagnostic criteria, highlighting the widespread and often underdiagnosed nature of the condition.

The Geographic Picture

Sleep apnea doesn't affect all regions equally. China, the United States, Brazil, and India have the highest absolute numbers of people with sleep apnea, partly due to their large populations. However, when we look at prevalence rates (the percentage of people affected), interesting patterns emerge that tell us sleep apnea isn't just about population size.

For example, in some countries with high obesity rates, like the United States, up to 17% of men and 9% of women have at least moderate sleep apnea. Meanwhile, despite lower obesity rates, some Asian populations show surprisingly high sleep apnea prevalence—often attributed to differences in facial structure and airway anatomy rather than body weight.

Did you know?

Recent studies show that ethnicity affects how sleep apnea manifests. African Americans tend to develop sleep apnea at younger ages than Caucasians, while Asians often develop sleep apnea at lower BMI levels due to differences in craniofacial structure, particularly having smaller maxillomandibular dimensions relative to body size.

This uneven global distribution points to complex interactions between genetics, lifestyle, and environment. Researchers studying these patterns have found that while obesity remains the strongest risk factor globally, its impact varies significantly across ethnic groups.

The Gender Gap

One of the most consistent findings across studies is that sleep apnea affects men more frequently than women—typically at a ratio of about 2-3 men for every woman diagnosed. This gender difference is especially pronounced during middle age.

Why this disparity? Several factors contribute:

- Hormonal differences: Female hormones, particularly progesterone, appear to protect women somewhat by increasing muscle tone in the upper airway and enhancing the brain's response to low oxygen levels.
- Fat distribution: Men tend to accumulate fat in the neck and torso (apple pattern), while women more often store fat in the hips and thighs (pear pattern). Neck fat directly increases pressure on the airway.
- Airway anatomy: Men generally have longer airways that are more vulnerable to collapse.

Interestingly, this gender gap narrows considerably after menopause, when women's hormone levels change. Post-menopausal women have rates of sleep apnea much closer to those of men, supporting the theory that female hormones play a protective role.

Research also suggests that diagnostic criteria may also contribute to this gender disparity. The Medicare 4% oxygen desaturation rule, which requires a 4% drop in oxygen levels to classify an event as sleep apnea, disproportionately excludes women from diagnosis and treatment. Women with sleep apnea tend to experience less severe oxygen desaturations but still suffer from symptoms like excessive daytime sleepiness, fatigue, and disrupted sleep.

A 2020 study found that using a 3% desaturation threshold instead of 4% increased OSA diagnoses by nearly 20%—many of whom were women who would otherwise go undiagnosed. This suggests that current definitions of sleep apnea may be biased toward how the condition presents in men, potentially leading to significant under-diagnosis and under-treatment of women.

However, in the last few years, there's been a strong push to close this gender gap in diagnosis and care. Notable developments include:

- Updated diagnostic criteria: Allowing hypopneas to be scored with a 3% oxygen drop or arousals helps capture more cases in women whose apneas may not cause deep desaturations.
- Better screening tools: New questionnaires and adjusted thresholds for neck circumference improve accuracy in identifying sleep apnea in women.
- Home testing: Wearable devices and home sleep tests are helping women access diagnosis more easily without the stigma or discomfort of lab-based studies.
- Awareness campaigns: Medical communities are increasingly educating providers to recognize sleep apnea symptoms in women beyond snoring.

These shifts have led to increased diagnosis rates in women and more inclusive treatment approaches. As the conversation broadens, women are getting the sleep health attention they long deserved.

The Age Factor

Sleep apnea prevalence increases dramatically with age. While the condition can affect people of any age (even children), the numbers climb steadily through adulthood:

- Among young adults (18-30), about 3-5% have significant sleep apnea.
- In middle age (30-60), rates increase to 10-17% for men and 3-9% for women.
- Among older adults (65+), the prevalence can exceed 30-40% in some studies.

Recent innovations are helping to close this age gap:

- Home testing for seniors: Simplified, portable devices allow older adults to be tested comfortably at home, avoiding complex lab setups.
- Tailored diagnostics: Modern algorithms detect shorter events and central apneas more common in older adults, even when oxygen levels don't drop dramatically.
- New tech for CSA: Devices like the FDA-approved *remedē System* stimulate the phrenic nerve to pace breathing during central apneas, especially in heart failure patients.

Health professionals are also shifting their views: sleep apnea treatment is now recognized as essential to preventing cognitive decline, strokes, and hospitalizations in seniors. Awareness campaigns and updated guidelines are encouraging routine screening of older adults during check-ups, helping them stay independent, alert, and healthy longer.

Identifying Symptoms

Sleep apnea often announces itself through a constellation of nighttime and daytime symptoms. Recognizing these warning signs is crucial, as they serve as important clues that should prompt further investigation.

Nighttime Warning Signs

The most recognizable nighttime symptoms of sleep apnea include:

- Loud, persistent snoring: While not everyone who snores has sleep apnea, nearly everyone with obstructive sleep apnea snores. The snoring is typically loud enough to be heard through walls or doors.
- Witnessed breathing pauses: Bed partners often report seeing the person stop breathing momentarily, followed by gasping, choking, or snorting as breathing resumes.
- Restless sleep: Tossing, turning, and frequent position changes throughout the night as the body tries to improve breathing.
- Nighttime awakenings: Many people with sleep apnea wake up multiple times during the night, often to use the bathroom (a symptom called nocturia).
- Night sweats: The body's stress response to breathing difficulties can trigger excessive sweating during sleep.

Did you know?

While loud snoring is present in about 85-90% of people with obstructive sleep apnea, it's much less common in central sleep apnea. This difference can provide an important clue about which type of sleep apnea someone might have. Additionally, research published in The Journal of Sleep Medicine and Disorders in 2016 found that women with sleep apnea tend to be lighter snorers than men, even when they have a significant sleep apnea burden. Because of this, many women with classic symptoms of sleep apnea may go undiagnosed if snoring is used as a primary diagnostic criterion.

Many of these nighttime symptoms go unnoticed by the person experiencing them. It's often a bed partner, roommate, or family member who first notices these concerning patterns. This is why sleep specialists often want to hear from someone who has observed the person sleeping.

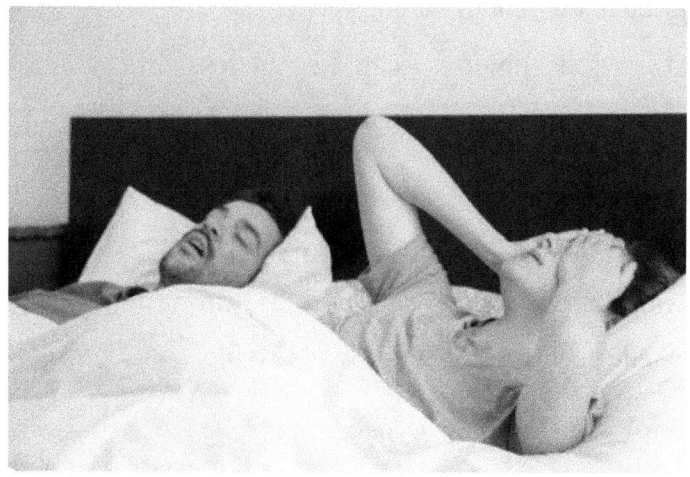

Loud, persistent snoring — another key symptom of sleep apnea. Photo credit: Pexels.

Daytime Consequences

The disrupted sleep caused by repeated breathing pauses leads to several daytime symptoms:

- Excessive daytime sleepiness: More than just feeling tired, this overwhelming drowsiness can make it difficult to stay awake during quiet activities.
- Morning headaches: Caused by oxygen deprivation and carbon dioxide buildup during the night.
- Difficulty concentrating: Problems with memory, attention, and mental clarity.
- Irritability and mood changes: Sleep disruption can cause significant mood disturbances, including symptoms that mimic depression and anxiety.
- Dry mouth or sore throat upon waking: Result of breathing through the mouth during sleep.
- Decreased libido: Reduced interest in sex, sometimes accompanied by erectile dysfunction in men.

These daytime symptoms can severely impact quality of life, work performance, and relationships. They also create safety concerns—people with untreated sleep apnea are 2-3 times more likely to have motor vehicle accidents due to drowsy driving.

How Symptoms Differ By Type

While there's considerable overlap, certain symptoms can help distinguish between the different types of sleep apnea. Recognizing these distinctions is essential for accurate diagnosis and targeted treatment, as each form of the condition has unique underlying mechanisms and associated risks.

Obstructive Sleep Apnea (OSA) typically presents with:

- Loud, chronic snoring, often punctuated by gasping or choking sounds
- Observable breathing interruptions, where the sleeper appears to stop breathing for several seconds before resuming
- Restless sleep, frequent awakenings, or a sensation of choking during the night
- Morning headaches due to oxygen deprivation and fluctuating carbon dioxide levels
- Excessive daytime sleepiness, difficulty concentrating, and irritability due to sleep fragmentation

Central Sleep Apnea (CSA) symptoms may include:

- Periods of paused breathing without the presence of snoring
- Shortness of breath upon waking
- Insomnia or difficulty maintaining sleep
- Daytime fatigue that is often unresponsive to typical interventions
- Symptoms of underlying conditions, such as heart failure or neurological disorders, which often coexist with CSA

Complex Sleep Apnea Syndrome (CompSA) symptoms may characterized by:

- Initial OSA symptoms, followed by persistent episodes of central apneas despite airway management
- Difficulty adapting to CPAP therapy
- Lingering fatigue and unrefreshing sleep, even with treatment

Understanding these symptoms is crucial for early detection and effective management of sleep apnea. Because untreated sleep apnea can contribute to serious health issues, including cardiovascular disease, cognitive decline, and metabolic disorders, prompt evaluation by a healthcare provider is recommended for individuals experiencing these symptoms.

Diagnosis through Sleep Studies

When David first visited his doctor complaining of constant fatigue despite sleeping eight hours each night, his wife mentioned his loud snoring and occasional gasping for air during sleep. These telltale signs prompted his doctor to recommend a sleep study—the definitive way to diagnose sleep apnea and determine its severity.

Sleep studies serve as the gold standard for diagnosing sleep apnea because they provide objective measurements of what happens to your breathing during sleep. Unlike many medical conditions that can be diagnosed through blood tests or physical examinations, sleep apnea requires monitoring of what happens when you're unconscious.

Sleep apnea isn't a one-size-fits-all condition. It comes in different types and severity levels, influenced by weight, anatomy, age, and lifestyle. This complexity means that even healthcare providers might miss key diagnostic details without proper testing.

Did you know?

A 2016 study by Chung et al. found that up to 90% of individuals with moderate-to-severe sleep apnea remain undiagnosed, underscoring how frequently this serious condition goes unrecognized without proper screening and testing.

Validated Screening Tools

Before diving into complex sleep studies, healthcare providers often use validated screening tools. These tools act as checkpoints to flag high-risk patients.

The Berlin Questionnaire: A Time-Tested Tool

The Berlin Questionnaire has been helping identify sleep apnea risk since 1996, making it one of the oldest and most widely used screening tools. It focuses on three key categories that paint a picture of your sleep apnea risk:

- Snoring behavior and sleep quality: Questions about snoring intensity, frequency, and whether you've been told you stop breathing during sleep
- Daytime sleepiness: How tired you feel during daily activities and whether you've ever nodded off while driving
- Hypertension and obesity: Your blood pressure history and body mass index (BMI)

If you score high in two or more categories, you're considered at high risk for sleep apnea. A 2017 review in the *Journal of Clinical Sleep Medicine* found that the Berlin Questionnaire catches about 76% of moderate to severe sleep apnea cases—not perfect, but an excellent starting point.

STOP-BANG: The Gold Standard for Surgical Patients

If you're considering sleep implant surgery, your healthcare team will likely use the STOP-BANG questionnaire. This tool was specifically designed to identify sleep apnea risk in surgical patients and has become the preferred screening method in pre-surgical evaluations.

STOP-BANG is an acronym that covers eight key risk factors:

- Snoring
- Tiredness during the day
- Observed apneas (has someone seen you stop breathing?)
- Pressure (high blood pressure)
- BMI over 35 kg/m²
- Age over 50
- Neck circumference larger than 40 cm (16 inches)
- Gender (male)

Each "yes" answer gives you one point. A score of 3 or more suggests increased risk, while five or more indicates a high risk for moderate to severe sleep apnea. What makes STOP-BANG particularly valuable is its high sensitivity—it rarely misses people who actually have sleep apnea, especially severe cases.

The Multi-Level Approach to Risk Assessment

Sleep specialists use a multi-level approach to categorize patients into different risk groups. This isn't just about putting people in boxes—it's about creating a roadmap for treatment that addresses each person's unique situation.

The stratification process typically follows these steps:

- Initial screening: Using questionnaires and basic measurements to identify those who need further testing
- Diagnostic testing: Confirming the presence and severity of sleep apnea
- Risk categorization: Classifying patients based on several factors
- Treatment matching: Determining the most appropriate intervention based on risk category

Key Categories in Sleep Apnea Stratification

When healthcare providers stratify sleep apnea patients, they typically place them into several key categories that guide treatment decisions:

Severity-Based Categories

These are based on the Apnea-Hypopnea Index (AHI) from sleep studies:

- Mild: AHI 5–15 events per hour
- Moderate: AHI 15–30 events per hour
- Severe: AHI greater than 30 events per hour

Treatment History Categories

- Treatment-naïve: Never treated

- CPAP-intolerant: Tried CPAP but couldn't adapt
- Treatment-resistant: Tried multiple therapies without success

Anatomical Categories

These are based on where the airway obstruction occurs:

- Tongue-based obstruction
- Palatal obstruction
- Multi-level obstruction

For patients considering sleep implants, these categories are crucial.

Choosing a Testing Method

There are two main methods for diagnosing sleep apnea:

Home Sleep Apnea Testing: Convenience and Accessibility

While laboratory testing provides the most detailed information, home sleep apnea tests (HSATs) have become increasingly popular. These portable devices allow you to sleep in your own bed while collecting essential data about your breathing patterns.

Home sleep tests typically measure:

- Airflow through a sensor under your nose
- Breathing effort via a belt around your chest
- Blood oxygen levels with a finger clip sensor
- Heart rate and sometimes position

More recently, newer ring-based home sleep test devices have been developed that measure the PPG (Photoplethysmography) signal from the finger. PPG technology allows for the continuous monitoring of blood flow variations, which can help detect changes in breathing and oxygen levels more accurately.

What home tests don't measure are brain waves, so they can't determine your sleep stages or exactly when you're asleep versus awake. This is their main limitation—they assume you're asleep during the entire recording period, which might not be accurate if you have insomnia or frequently wake up.

Home testing works best for patients with a high probability of moderate to severe obstructive sleep apnea who don't have other significant medical conditions. They're particularly useful for people who can't easily travel to a sleep lab, feel anxious about sleeping in an unfamiliar environment, or have mobility issues.

In-Lab Polysomnography: The Gold Standard

The most comprehensive sleep study is called polysomnography (PSG), typically conducted in a specialized sleep laboratory. During this test, you'll spend the night in a private room that resembles a hotel room more than a hospital setting. A sleep technologist will attach various sensors to monitor multiple body functions while you sleep.

These sensors track:

- Brain waves through electrodes placed on your scalp that show your sleep stages and how often you wake
- Eye movements to identify REM (rapid eye movement) sleep

- Heart rhythm via electrocardiogram (ECG) leads
- Muscle activity in your chin and legs
- Airflow through your nose and mouth
- Breathing effort from chest and abdominal bands
- Blood oxygen levels using a fingertip or earlobe sensor
- Body position to see if sleep apnea worsens when you lie on your back

Did you know?

The simultaneous measurement of airflow and breathing effort is what allows sleep specialists to distinguish between obstructive and central sleep apnea. In obstructive events, the chest and abdomen continue moving (showing effort) despite blocked airflow, while in central events, both airflow and breathing effort cease simultaneously.

What makes in-lab polysomnography particularly valuable is the presence of a trained technologist who can observe your sleep directly and make adjustments if sensors come loose. They can also document unusual behaviors like sleepwalking or acting out dreams that might indicate other sleep disorders.

Limitations of In-Lab Sleep Studies

Despite being the gold standard, in-lab sleep studies aren't without their downsides. For many patients, the experience can be uncomfortable, intimidating, or even inaccessible.

- Unnatural sleep environment: Trying to fall asleep while hooked up to wires in an unfamiliar setting can affect how you sleep—possibly skewing the results.
- Cost and insurance: Polysomnography can be expensive, and not all insurance plans cover it fully. This financial barrier may prevent some people from seeking a diagnosis.
- Limited availability: In some regions, long wait times for in-lab studies can delay diagnosis and treatment.

These limitations don't make in-lab studies any less important—but they do highlight why home sleep testing and newer wearable technologies are becoming valuable tools, especially for initial screenings or follow-up monitoring.

Cardiovascular Risk and Complications

Sleep apnea doesn't just rob you of restful sleep—it puts extraordinary stress on your heart and blood vessels. This makes it a significant risk factor for serious cardiovascular problems, often operating silently until damage has accumulated over the years.

The Nightly Cardiovascular Roller Coaster

To understand why sleep apnea is so damaging to your cardiovascular system, imagine what happens during each breathing pause:

- As your airway closes or your brain fails to signal breathing, oxygen levels in your blood begin to drop.

- Your brain detects this dangerous situation and triggers a "fight or flight" stress response.
- Your sympathetic nervous system floods your body with stress hormones like adrenaline.
- Your heart rate spikes and blood vessels constrict, causing blood pressure to surge.
- This stress response partially awakens you, restoring breathing but fragmenting your sleep.

Now imagine this cycle happening dozens or even hundreds of times each night, night after night. Your cardiovascular system never gets the rest it needs during sleep—instead, it's repeatedly subjected to surges of stress hormones, pressure changes, and oxygen deprivation.

Did you know?

During sleep apnea episodes, blood pressure can spike by 20-30 mmHg or more. For someone with moderate to severe sleep apnea, these surges can occur 30+ times per hour. This creates a "non-dipping" blood pressure pattern where pressure stays elevated throughout the night instead of naturally decreasing during sleep as it should.

Hypertension: The Silent Connection

One of the most well-established links between sleep apnea and cardiovascular health is hypertension (high blood pressure). Research shows that approximately 50% of people with sleep apnea develop hypertension, and conversely, about 30% of people with hypertension have sleep apnea—often undiagnosed.

Sleep apnea doesn't just cause temporary blood pressure spikes during sleep; it leads to persistent daytime hypertension as well. This happens because the repeated stress responses reset your body's blood pressure regulation systems to a higher level. Even more concerning, sleep apnea is a common cause of resistant hypertension—high blood pressure that remains uncontrolled despite multiple medications.

The relationship is so strong that the American Heart Association recommends sleep apnea screening for people with hypertension, particularly those whose blood pressure is difficult to control with standard treatments. If you have high blood pressure that isn't responding well to medication, consider asking your heart doctor whether sleep apnea testing might be right for you. Identifying and treating an underlying sleep disorder could be a key step in better managing your blood pressure and overall cardiovascular health.

Heart Disease and Stroke Risk

Beyond hypertension, untreated sleep apnea significantly increases your risk of other serious cardiovascular problems:

- Coronary Artery Disease: The repeated oxygen drops and stress responses damage the lining of blood vessels and promote inflammation, accelerating the buildup of plaque in coronary arteries. Studies show people with severe sleep apnea have a 2-3 times higher risk of heart disease.
- Heart Failure: The strain of working against elevated pressure night after night can cause your heart muscle to thicken and

weaken over time. Sleep apnea is particularly common in people with heart failure, creating a dangerous cycle where each condition worsens the other.
- Arrhythmias: Sleep apnea increases the risk of irregular heartbeats, especially atrial fibrillation (AFib). During apnea episodes, the heart's electrical system becomes unstable due to oxygen fluctuations and heightened sympathetic activity.

Neurological and Cognitive Effects

The brain is particularly vulnerable to the effects of sleep apnea. While we often focus on the cardiovascular complications, the neurological and cognitive impacts can be equally devastating, affecting everything from daily functioning to long-term brain health.

The Oxygen Deprivation Cascade

Each time breathing stops during a sleep apnea episode, oxygen levels in the blood drop. The brain, which consumes about 20% of the body's oxygen despite making up only 2% of body weight, is extremely sensitive to these fluctuations. This repeated oxygen deprivation, called intermittent hypoxia, triggers a cascade of harmful processes:

- Oxidative stress damages brain cells through the release of harmful free radicals
- Inflammation increases throughout brain tissue
- Blood-brain barrier function becomes compromised

- Neurotransmitter systems that regulate mood and cognition become dysregulated

Beyond the direct effects of oxygen deprivation, sleep apnea fragments sleep and prevents the deep, restorative stages that are crucial for brain maintenance. During healthy deep sleep, the brain clears away waste products, consolidates memories, and performs essential "maintenance" functions. Sleep apnea disrupts these processes, leading to a brain that's essentially running on emergency power.

Did you know?

Recent research using brain imaging has shown that untreated sleep apnea leads to reductions in both gray and white matter volume, particularly in regions linked to memory and attention. A 2016 study published by the American Academy of Sleep Medicine found that severe sleep apnea was associated with widespread white matter damage. However, after 12 months of CPAP therapy, these abnormalities largely reversed, alongside improvements in cognitive function and alertness. This highlights the brain's ability to recover with proper oxygenation and restorative sleep.

Everyday Cognitive Challenges

For many people with sleep apnea, cognitive difficulties are among the most frustrating daily symptoms. These typically include:

- Attention and concentration problems: Difficulty focusing on tasks, being easily distracted, and struggling to maintain attention during conversations or meetings

- Memory impairment: Forgetting appointments, misplacing items, or having trouble learning and retaining new information
- Executive function deficits: Challenges with planning, organizing, problem-solving, and multitasking
- Slowed thinking and reaction time: Taking longer to process information and respond appropriately
- Mental flexibility issues: Difficulty adapting to changing situations or shifting between tasks

These cognitive effects can be particularly devastating in professional settings. Many people with untreated sleep apnea report declining work performance, missing deadlines, and making errors they would have easily caught before. For students, learning becomes more challenging, and academic performance may suffer.

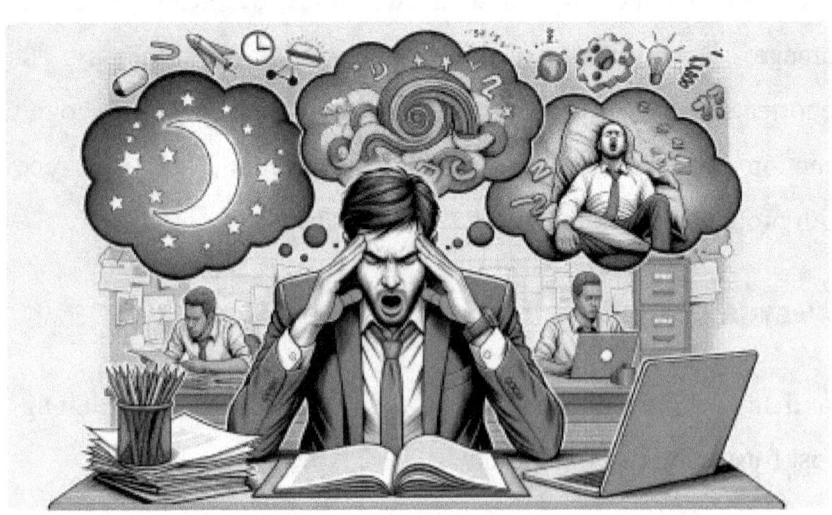

Illustration: Cognitive effects of sleep apnea on daily tasks.

Emotional and Psychological Impact

The brain changes caused by sleep apnea don't just affect thinking—they also influence mood, emotional regulation, and overall mental well-being. The chronic sleep disruption and oxygen deprivation caused by sleep apnea can create a perfect storm for psychological distress.

- Irritability and mood swings: Quick to anger, easily frustrated, and often emotionally volatile
- Depression symptoms: Persistent low mood, loss of interest in activities, fatigue, and feelings of hopelessness or worthlessness
- Anxiety: Elevated heart rate, racing thoughts, and panic attacks are not uncommon, especially when breathing difficulties disrupt sleep cycles
- Emotional numbness: Some individuals report feeling emotionally "flat," unable to enjoy life or connect with others

These symptoms are not simply side effects of poor sleep—they're signs of the brain struggling under the cumulative stress of disrupted oxygen flow and chronic sleep fragmentation. Over time, the effects of untreated sleep apnea can mimic major depressive disorder or generalized anxiety disorder, leading to misdiagnosis if sleep health isn't assessed.

The emotional toll of sleep apnea also extends into relationships and quality of life. Mood instability and excessive daytime sleepiness can make it hard to maintain social connections, fulfill parenting responsibilities, or engage meaningfully with partners and friends. Over time, this social withdrawal can worsen feelings of isolation and sadness.

Fortunately, the emotional effects of sleep apnea are often reversible. Many people find that once their sleep is properly treated, their mood stabilizes, anxiety subsides, and they begin to feel like themselves again. Restorative sleep truly is a foundational element of emotional health.

Metabolic and Hormonal Impact

Sleep apnea doesn't just affect your breathing and sleep quality—it fundamentally disrupts your body's metabolic and hormonal balance. This disruption creates a dangerous cycle where sleep apnea contributes to metabolic disorders, which then worsen sleep apnea.

The Insulin Resistance Connection

One of the most significant metabolic effects of sleep apnea is insulin resistance—a condition where your cells don't respond properly to insulin, the hormone that regulates blood sugar. During sleep apnea episodes, your oxygen levels repeatedly drop and rise, creating what scientists call "intermittent hypoxia."

This oxygen roller coaster triggers several harmful processes:

- Your body releases stress hormones like cortisol and adrenaline
- Inflammation increases throughout your tissues

- Your liver increases glucose production
- Muscle and fat cells become less responsive to insulin

The result? Your blood sugar levels rise, and your pancreas must produce more insulin to compensate. Over time, this strain can lead to insulin resistance and eventually type 2 diabetes. Studies show that moderate to severe sleep apnea increases diabetes risk by 30% or more, even after accounting for obesity.

Did you know?

A single night of fragmented sleep can reduce insulin sensitivity by 25% in otherwise healthy adults. For someone with sleep apnea experiencing disrupted sleep every night for years, the cumulative impact on glucose metabolism can be profound, explaining why treating sleep apnea often improves blood sugar control in diabetic patients.

Hunger Hormones Gone Haywire

Have you ever noticed that when you're tired, you crave carbohydrates and high-calorie foods? This isn't just a lack of willpower—it's your hormones at work. Sleep apnea significantly disrupts the delicate balance of hormones that regulate hunger and fullness:

- Leptin, your "fullness hormone," decreases with sleep apnea, making you feel less satisfied after eating
- Ghrelin, your "hunger hormone," increases, stimulating appetite and cravings, particularly for high-carbohydrate foods

- GLP-1 (glucagon-like peptide-1), which helps you feel full and regulates insulin, becomes dysregulated

This hormonal chaos creates the perfect storm for weight gain. People with untreated sleep apnea often find themselves in a frustrating cycle—they gain weight despite their best efforts at diet and exercise, and this additional weight worsens their sleep apnea, further disrupting their hormones.

The Metabolic Syndrome Connection

Sleep apnea is strongly linked to metabolic syndrome—a cluster of conditions that occur together, increasing your risk of heart disease, stroke, and diabetes. These conditions include:

- Increased blood pressure
- High blood sugar
- Excess body fat around the waist
- Abnormal cholesterol level

This interconnectedness shows how crucial it is to address sleep apnea not only for better sleep but also for overall metabolic health.

Athletic Performance and Sleep Apnea

Whether you're a weekend warrior or a professional competitor, the quality of your sleep directly affects how well you perform. For athletes with undiagnosed sleep apnea, that relationship becomes a significant barrier to reaching their potential.

When we exercise, especially at high intensities, we create microscopic damage to muscle fibers. This damage isn't harmful—in fact, it's necessary for improvement. During sleep, particularly deep sleep, the body repairs this damage, building muscles back stronger than before. Growth hormone, which peaks during deep sleep, plays a crucial role in this recovery process.

For athletes with sleep apnea, this essential recovery cycle gets hijacked. Each time breathing stops, oxygen levels drop, and the body shifts into survival mode. The resulting stress response and sleep fragmentation dramatically reduce time spent in deep sleep—precisely when muscle recovery should be happening.

Did you know?

Athletes with untreated sleep apnea show up to 30% lower nighttime growth hormone secretion compared to their healthy counterparts. Since growth hormone is essential for muscle repair and development, this deficiency directly impacts recovery time and training adaptations.

The consequences are predictable but often misinterpreted: persistent muscle soreness, increased injury risk, and diminished training responses. Many athletes mistake these symptoms for overtraining and respond by pushing harder—creating a destructive cycle that further depletes their already compromised recovery capacity.

Endurance under Siege

Endurance athletes rely on their cardiovascular system's efficiency to deliver oxygen to working muscles. Sleep apnea undermines this system in multiple ways:

- Reduced oxygen efficiency: Repeated episodes of low oxygen during sleep can decrease the body's ability to utilize oxygen effectively during exercise.
- Impaired cardiac function: The strain sleep apnea places on the heart reduces cardiac output—the amount of blood your heart can pump per minute.
- Chronic inflammation: Sleep apnea triggers inflammatory responses that can impair blood vessel function and reduce aerobic capacity.
- Energy depletion: The constant arousal and stress responses during sleep consume energy resources that would otherwise be available during training or competition.

These effects explain why athletes with sleep apnea often hit their "wall" much earlier than expected. Their perceived exertion feels higher at lower workloads, and recovery between intervals takes longer. What's particularly insidious is that many endurance athletes attribute this decline to aging or insufficient training rather than a treatable sleep disorder.

Reaction Time and Decision-Making

In sports requiring quick reactions and tactical decisions—from tennis to team sports like basketball or soccer—cognitive sharpness is as important as physical ability. Athletes must process information rapidly, anticipate opponents' moves, and execute precise actions under pressure. Sleep apnea impairs these mental aspects of performance through several mechanisms, affecting both reaction speed and decision-making efficiency.

- Slowed reaction time: Studies indicate that reaction time can decrease by up to 10-20% in people with moderate to severe sleep apnea. This decline results from fragmented sleep, leading to deficits in alertness and motor coordination. Even microseconds of delay can be detrimental in high-speed sports, where split-second decisions determine success or failure.
- Impaired decision-making: The ability to process information quickly and make strategic choices diminishes with sleep fragmentation. Athletes with untreated sleep apnea often struggle with situational awareness, problem-solving, and response inhibition—critical skills for adjusting tactics in real time and avoiding errors.
- Reduced focus and concentration: The cognitive burden of sleep deprivation impairs sustained attention, increasing the likelihood of lapses in concentration. This can lead to mistakes in high-stakes moments, whether it's a misjudged pass, a

delayed sprint, or a failure to anticipate an opponent's movement.

- Increased risk of injury: Impaired reflexes and delayed reaction times heighten the risk of on-field injuries. Athletes with sleep apnea may be slower to brace for impact, avoid collisions, or maintain proper body mechanics during complex maneuvers.

These cognitive deficits can have long-term consequences, not only reducing athletic performance but also increasing susceptibility to mental fatigue and burnout. Addressing sleep apnea through proper diagnosis and treatment—such as CPAP therapy, lifestyle adjustments, and optimizing sleep hygiene—can help restore cognitive sharpness, allowing athletes to perform at their peak both mentally and physically.

CPAP Therapy Overview

Imagine this: you're lying in bed, eyes closed, seemingly asleep. But inside your body, a silent battle rages as your airway repeatedly collapses, forcing you to briefly wake dozens—sometimes hundreds—of times throughout the night. This is the reality for millions with sleep apnea. For decades, one treatment has stood as the frontline defense against this exhausting condition: CPAP therapy.

CPAP, which stands for Continuous Positive Airway Pressure, has been the gold standard treatment for sleep apnea since the early 1980s. But what exactly is this device that many compare to Darth Vader's mask, and how does it help people breathe better at night?

How CPAP Works: A Gentle Air Splint

At its core, CPAP therapy is brilliantly simple: it delivers a constant stream of pressurized air through a mask worn over your nose or mouth while you sleep. This pressurized air acts like an invisible splint, holding your airway open and preventing it from collapsing.

Think of your airway as a soft, flexible tube. In people with obstructive sleep apnea, the muscles supporting this tube relax too much during sleep, causing it to narrow or collapse completely. The CPAP machine counteracts this by pushing just enough air pressure to keep the tube open—like inflating a balloon just enough to maintain its shape without overinflating it.

Did you know?

CPAP works immediately to reduce apnea events. Many patients report feeling more refreshed after just one night of use, though it typically takes 2 to 3 weeks of consistent use to experience the full benefits of improved daytime alertness and reduced fatigue.

This continuous pressure ensures that your airway remains open throughout the entire breathing cycle—both when you breathe in and when you breathe out. This distinguishes CPAP from natural breathing, where the pressure in the airway fluctuates between inhalation and exhalation.

The Components of a CPAP System

A typical CPAP setup consists of three main components:

- The machine: A small, quiet air compressor that draws in room air, filters it, and pressurizes it to the prescribed setting
- The tubing: A lightweight, flexible hose that carries the pressurized air from the machine to the mask
- The mask: Available in various styles (nasal pillows, nasal masks, or full-face masks) to suit different facial structures and breathing patterns

Modern CPAP machines often include additional features that enhance comfort and effectiveness. Many have built-in humidifiers to prevent dryness in the nose and throat. Others offer "ramp" features that start with lower pressure and gradually increase to the prescribed level as you fall asleep. Some of the newest models even automatically adjust pressure throughout the night based on your breathing patterns.

Effectiveness: The Numbers Tell the Story

When it comes to treating obstructive sleep apnea, CPAP's effectiveness is remarkable. Studies consistently show that proper CPAP use can:

- Reduce the Apnea-Hypopnea Index (AHI)—the number of breathing interruptions per hour—by 90% or more in many patients
- Increase blood oxygen levels during sleep to normal ranges
- Significantly reduce daytime sleepiness and fatigue
- Lower blood pressure, particularly nighttime blood pressure
- Improve concentration, mood, and overall quality of life

Challenges and Compliance Issues

Despite its effectiveness, CPAP therapy faces a significant hurdle: many people simply don't use it consistently enough to reap the benefits. Studies show that 30-50% of patients either abandon CPAP therapy entirely or use it far less than the recommended amount (at least four hours per night on 70% of nights).

This low adherence rate isn't simply a matter of patient stubbornness or lack of motivation. Multiple factors contribute to what sleep specialists call "the compliance conundrum."

Did you know?

Research shows that a patient's experience during the first week of CPAP use strongly predicts long-term adherence. Those who use their CPAP for at least 4 hours per night during the first week are much more likely to become consistent users. This highlights the critical importance of addressing comfort and adaptation issues early in treatment.

Physical Discomfort and Mask Issues

For many patients, physical discomfort presents the most immediate barrier to CPAP use. Common complaints include:

- Mask discomfort: Pressure points, skin irritation, and facial marks from mask straps and cushions
- Air leaks: Gaps between the mask and face that cause annoying air jets and reduce therapy effectiveness

- Pressure intolerance: Difficulty exhaling against the incoming air pressure, creating a sensation of fighting against the machine
- Nasal congestion and dryness: Irritation of nasal passages from airflow, particularly in dry climates or heated homes
- Noise disturbances: Machine sounds that disturb either the user or their bed partner

Psychological and Emotional Barriers

Beyond physical discomfort, many patients face psychological hurdles that can be even more challenging to overcome:

- Claustrophobia: The sensation of having something covering the face can trigger anxiety and panic in some users
- Self-image concerns: Feeling unattractive or embarrassed wearing the device, particularly in front of partners
- Frustration with complexity: Difficulty managing the equipment, especially for older adults or those with limited dexterity
- Sleep anxiety: Paradoxically developing worry about sleep itself, which makes relaxation more difficult

These psychological factors often interact with personality traits. Research by Maschauer and colleagues found that certain personality types—particularly those with high anxiety or hypochondriacal tendencies—tend to have lower CPAP compliance rates.

Conclusion and Transition

Throughout this chapter, we've taken a deep dive into the world of sleep apnea—a condition that affects nearly one billion adults worldwide and disrupts far more than just your night's rest. We've explored how this disorder manifests in its various forms: the airway collapses in obstructive sleep apnea, the brain fails to send proper breathing signals in central sleep apnea, or a complex combination of both occurs in some patients.

We've seen how sleep apnea isn't just about snoring or feeling tired—it's a serious health condition with far-reaching consequences. From cardiovascular risks like hypertension and heart disease to cognitive impairments, metabolic disruptions, and even decreased athletic performance, untreated sleep apnea affects virtually every system in your body.

This brings us to the exciting frontier of sleep apnea treatment—a landscape that has expanded dramatically in recent years. While CPAP remains valuable for many patients, the medical community now recognizes the importance of having multiple treatment approaches available to address the diverse needs of sleep apnea sufferers.

Looking forward to Chapter 2, we'll step into the fascinating world of medical innovation to uncover how sleep implants came to be. From the early breakthroughs in sleep apnea research to the engineering challenges behind modern neurostimulation devices, this next chapter will reveal the science and evolution behind these life-changing technologies—and how they're offering new hope to patients who struggle with traditional treatments like CPAP.

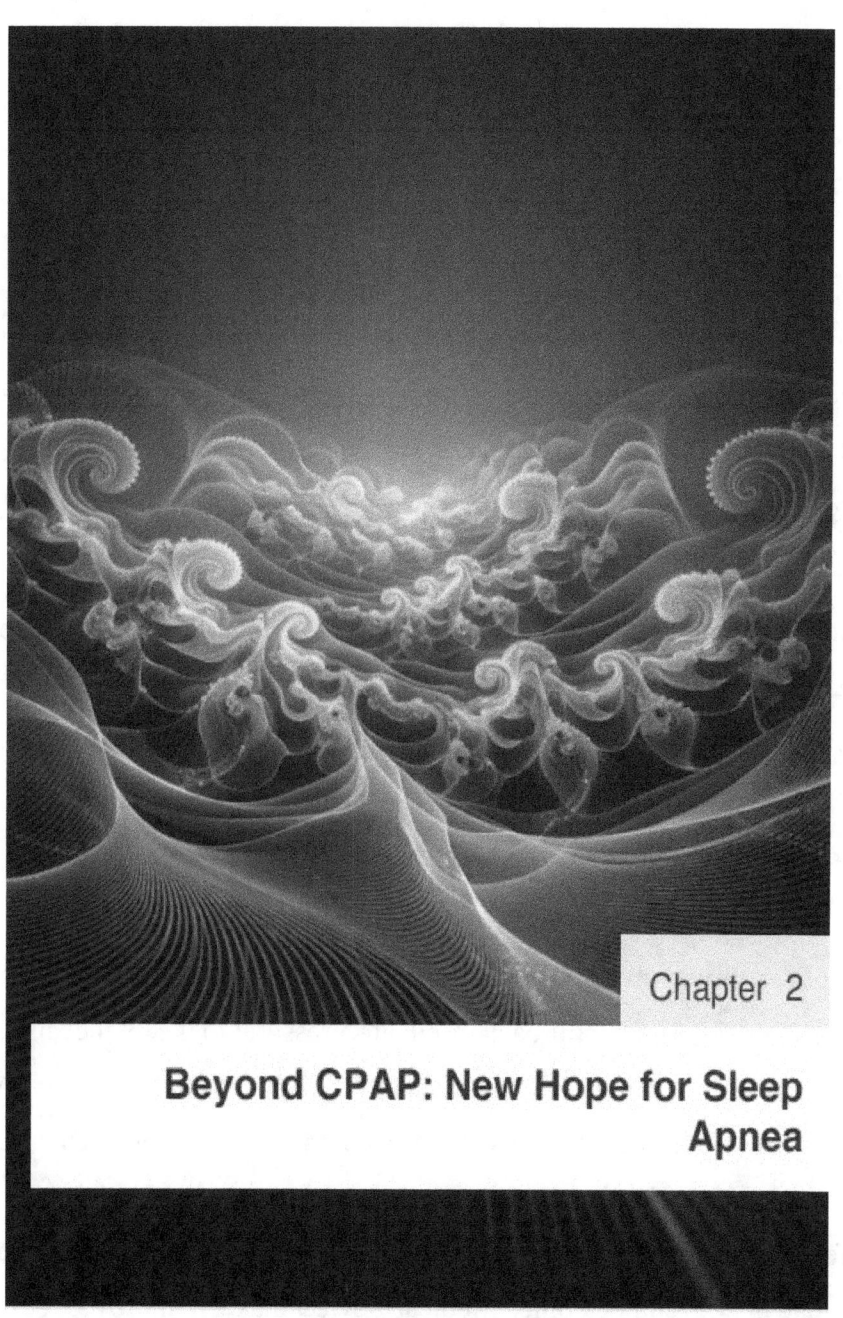

Chapter 2

Beyond CPAP: New Hope for Sleep Apnea

Chapter 2:
The Science behind Sleep Implants

Historical Development of Sleep Implants

The journey from early ideas to today's sophisticated sleep implants reads like a medical detective story—one where researchers, doctors, and engineers joined forces to tackle the stubborn problem of sleep apnea when traditional treatments fell short.

Our story begins in the 1970s when sleep medicine was still finding its footing. Researchers had just begun to understand that many people stopped breathing repeatedly during sleep—a condition we now know as sleep apnea. At first, doctors thought this was simply a quirky sleep behavior. But as evidence mounted showing connections to heart problems, strokes, and even early death, the search for effective treatments gained urgency.

The first breakthrough came in 1981 when Australian researcher Dr. Colin Sullivan invented continuous positive airway pressure (CPAP). This revolutionary approach used air pressure to keep the airway open—like inflating a collapsed tent from the inside. While CPAP worked wonderfully when used properly, a stubborn problem emerged: many patients simply couldn't tolerate wearing a mask all night. Some felt claustrophobic, others developed skin irritation, and many just found it too cumbersome. Medical device makers improved CPAP machines over time—making them smaller, quieter, and more comfortable—but compliance remained a significant hurdle.

Did you know?

Studies have shown that CPAP adherence declines over time, making long-term use a challenge for many patients. A 2023 study in BMC Pulmonary Medicine found that only 25.7% of first-time CPAP users with mild obstructive sleep apnea remained adherent after 12 months. This is particularly concerning given the crucial role that consistent CPAP use plays in reducing the risks associated with untreated sleep apnea, such as cardiovascular disease, stroke, and daytime fatigue. Similarly, a 2025 study in Thorax reported that 62% of patients were non-adherent by the third month, with early non-adherence strongly predicting long-term discontinuation. This early drop-off in adherence is particularly problematic, as studies have shown that the first few months of therapy are critical in establishing consistent usage patterns. While initial adherence rates may seem promising, these findings highlight a significant decline over time, underscoring the need for more effective, patient-centered interventions. Potential strategies could include alternative treatments, such as positional therapy, oral appliances, or surgical interventions for select cases. Additionally, personalized support strategies—such as regular follow-up appointments, patient education, and the use of digital tools like mobile apps to track usage—could help to mitigate the adherence gap and ensure better long-term management of sleep apnea.

Meanwhile, scientists were exploring the physiology of sleep apnea more deeply. In 1978, researcher John Remmers and colleagues made a crucial discovery: during sleep, the tongue's main muscle (the genioglossus) relaxes, allowing the tongue to fall backward and block the airway. This insight sparked a question: What if we could keep that muscle active during sleep?

Early experiments in the 1980s tried using electrical stimulation on the tongue muscles directly. While this showed promise in keeping airways open, it had a major flaw—the stimulation was strong enough to wake patients up! Clearly, a more refined approach was needed.

The next leap forward came when researchers shifted focus to stimulating the hypoglossal nerve—the nerve that controls the tongue—rather than the tongue muscle itself. This allowed for more precise control with less disruption to sleep. By the early 2000s, the concept of an implantable "pacemaker for the tongue" began to take shape.

The road to creating a viable implant wasn't smooth. Engineers had to solve numerous challenges: How to detect when a person was breathing in? How to deliver just the right amount of stimulation? How to make a device that would last for years inside the body? And most importantly, how to ensure it wouldn't disrupt sleep while preventing apneas?

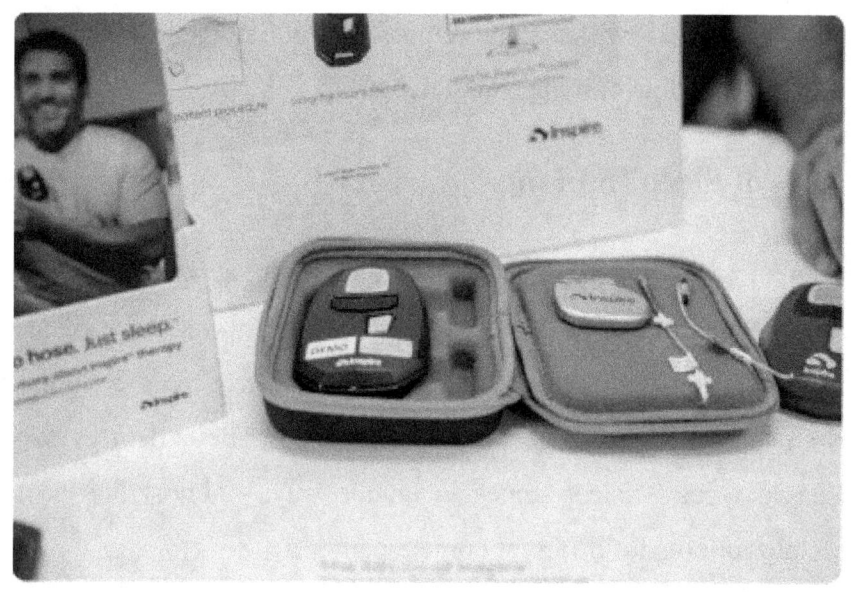

Inspire™ Upper Airway Stimulation

Inspire™ Upper Airway Stimulation

After years of development and clinical testing, a breakthrough came in 2014 when the Inspire™ Upper Airway Stimulation device became the first sleep implant to receive FDA approval for treating obstructive sleep apnea (OSA) in patients who couldn't tolerate CPAP. This approval was based on the STAR trial (Stimulation Therapy for Apnea Reduction), a pivotal study that demonstrated a 70% reduction in apnea events and marked improvements in daytime functioning and sleep quality. The success of this study helped establish hypoglossal nerve stimulation (HNS) as a viable alternative for CPAP-intolerant patients.

The Inspire system works by monitoring breathing patterns and delivering mild stimulation to the hypoglossal nerve with each breath, causing the tongue to move slightly forward and opening the airway.

Patients activate it with a small remote control before sleep and turn it off in the morning—no mask required.

Types of Sleep Implants

When most people think about treating sleep apnea, they picture someone wearing a CPAP mask. But beneath the surface of sleep medicine lies a fascinating world of implantable devices designed to help people breathe easier while they sleep. These devices target different types of sleep apnea in unique ways—almost like having specialized tools for different home repairs.

Let's explore the main categories of sleep implants and discover how each one tackles specific breathing challenges during sleep.

Hypoglossal Nerve Stimulation (HNS) Implants

Hypoglossal nerve stimulation implants are widely considered as having a pacemaker but for your tongue. HNS implants are designed specifically for obstructive sleep apnea (OSA) and include three main parts: a small pulse generator (about the size of a matchbox) implanted in the upper chest, a breathing sensor placed between the ribs, and a stimulation lead connected to the hypoglossal nerve—the nerve that controls your tongue movements.

When you're sleeping, the sensor detects your breathing pattern. Each time you inhale, the device sends a gentle electrical pulse to your hypoglossal nerve, causing your tongue to move slightly forward. This simple action keeps your airway open, preventing the blockage that causes obstructive sleep apnea.

Did you know?

A systematic review of 44 studies involving 8,670 patients found that hypoglossal nerve stimulation significantly improved sleep apnea outcomes, with 72% of patients achieving an apnea-hypopnea index (AHI) of less than ten after 12 months. Clinical success rates were reported at 80% within the first year. Additionally, improvements in quality of life scores suggest patients experienced better overall well-being post-treatment.

The most well-known HNS device is the Inspire™ system, which received FDA approval in 2014. Since then, other manufacturers have developed their own versions, each with slight variations in design and functionality.

Phrenic Nerve Stimulation Systems

While HNS devices target obstructive sleep apnea, phrenic nerve stimulators address a different condition: central sleep apnea (CSA). Remember from Chapter 1 that CSA occurs when your brain temporarily fails to send proper signals to the breathing muscles—it's not about blockage but about the breathing "command center" taking unwanted breaks.

The Remedē® System is the primary phrenic nerve stimulator approved for treating central sleep apnea. Instead of targeting the tongue, this device stimulates the phrenic nerve, which controls the diaphragm—your primary breathing muscle.

The Remedē system includes a small generator implanted in the chest and thin wires (leads) that are threaded through veins to sit near the phrenic nerve. Unlike HNS, which works with each breath, the phrenic stimulator monitors breathing patterns and only activates when it detects an abnormal pause—making it perfect for the intermittent nature of central sleep apnea.

Emerging Implant Technologies

Beyond these established systems, researchers are developing innovative approaches to treating sleep apnea with implantable devices.

One fascinating example is the development of "smart" polymer implants. These small, flexible devices can be placed in the soft palate or tongue base to provide structural support to prevent collapse. Some experimental versions even respond to magnetic fields, allowing external control of airway positioning without continuous electrical stimulation.

Another approach involves targeted muscle retraining through implanted electrodes that stimulate multiple airway muscles simultaneously. This "multi-site" stimulation aims to provide more comprehensive airway support than single-nerve stimulation.

Technical Anatomy of Sleep Implants

If you've ever wondered what exactly is inside those remarkable devices that help people breathe better while sleeping, you're about to find out. Let's take a peek under the hood of modern sleep implants and discover the ingenious components that make them work.

Think of a sleep implant as a symphony of specialized parts working in perfect harmony. Each component plays a crucial role in helping you breathe freely throughout the night. Using the hypoglossal nerve stimulator as our model (the most common sleep implant), let's explore the three main components that make this technology possible.

The Pulse Generator: The Brain of the Operation

The pulse generator is the command center of the entire system—essentially a small computer with a battery. About the size of a small matchbox, this flat, rounded device is typically implanted under the skin just below your collarbone.

Inside its titanium casing (chosen for durability and biocompatibility), the pulse generator houses a battery designed to last 8-11 years. When it eventually runs low, a relatively simple outpatient procedure allows doctors to replace just the generator while leaving the other components in place.

The generator creates precisely calibrated electrical pulses—mild enough not to disturb your sleep but strong enough to activate the tongue muscles that keep your airway open. It's also programmed with customized settings determined during your "titration" sessions with your sleep doctor.

The Breathing Sensor: Your Sleep's Vigilant Guardian

For a sleep implant to work effectively, it needs to know exactly when you're breathing in. That's where the breathing sensor (sometimes called the "sensing lead") comes into play.

This thin, flexible wire is carefully positioned between your ribs to monitor your breathing pattern. With each breath you take, your chest expands and contracts, creating subtle pressure changes that the sensor detects.

When the sensor detects you're beginning to inhale, it immediately signals the pulse generator to send a stimulation pulse. This perfect timing ensures your tongue moves forward precisely when you need your airway to be open.

In some newer models, this sensing function has been integrated directly into the pulse generator, eliminating the need for a separate sensor lead. This advancement simplifies the implantation procedure and reduces potential complications.

The Stimulation Lead: The Vital Connection

The third crucial component is the stimulation lead—a specialized wire with an electrode cuff at the end. This lead connects the pulse generator to the hypoglossal nerve under your tongue.

The electrode cuff is a marvel of biomedical engineering. Shaped like a small, flexible collar, it wraps partially around the hypoglossal nerve without compressing it. This design allows it to deliver electrical stimulation while minimizing the risk of nerve damage.

This selective stimulation is crucial—it ensures your tongue moves in a way that opens your airway rather than potentially making the obstruction worse. During surgery, doctors carefully test the response to find the optimal placement.

Design Considerations in Sleep Implants

Creating a device that lives inside the human body and functions reliably for years while you sleep presents fascinating engineering challenges. Sleep implants must balance effectiveness, safety, and user comfort—all while operating in the complex environment of the human body. Let's explore the key design considerations that engineers and medical device creators must address when developing these remarkable devices.

Biocompatibility: Making Friends with the Body

Perhaps the most fundamental challenge in designing any implantable device is ensuring the body accepts it as a non-threatening presence. For sleep implants, this means selecting materials that won't cause inflammation, allergic reactions, or tissue damage over many years. Modern devices typically use medical-grade titanium for outer casings, platinum-iridium alloys for electrodes, and specially formulated silicone or polyurethane for insulation and flexible components.

Engineers must also consider the physical interface between the device and surrounding tissues. The nerve cuff that wraps around the hypoglossal nerve, for instance, must make sufficient contact for electrical stimulation without causing pressure damage or restricting blood flow to the nerve.

Power Efficiency: The Battery Life Challenge

Unlike your smartphone that you can plug in each night, a sleep implant must operate for years on a single battery. This creates an intense focus on power efficiency in every aspect of the design.

The stimulation patterns are carefully calibrated to use just enough energy to activate the targeted muscles without waste. Modern implants also incorporate smart power management—for example, shutting down most functions during the day when therapy isn't needed or varying stimulation intensity based on sleep position or breathing patterns.

Battery technology itself presents unique challenges. The batteries must be completely sealed to prevent leakage, maintain stable output over the years, and be as energy-dense as possible while remaining safe. Most current sleep implants use lithium-based batteries similar to those in cardiac pacemakers, providing 8-11 years of nightly use before requiring replacement.

Size and Ergonomics: The Comfort Factor

While early medical implants prioritized function over form, modern sleep implants must be designed with patient comfort in mind. This means creating devices that are as small and unobtrusive as possible while still delivering effective therapy.

Engineers work to create pulse generators with rounded edges and slim profiles that sit comfortably under the skin. The placement locations—

typically below the collarbone for the generator and between ribs for sensors—are chosen to minimize movement and pressure during sleep and daily activities.

The leads (wires) connecting components must be flexible enough to move with the body without creating tension or discomfort yet durable enough to withstand millions of movement cycles over years of use. This often involves specialized materials and strain-relief designs at connection points.

Efficacy Studies: Sleep Implants vs. CPAP

When we talk about treating sleep apnea, the million-dollar question is simple: "Does it work?" For decades, CPAP has been the gold standard treatment, but sleep implants have emerged as an exciting alternative. Let's dive into what the research actually tells us about how these two approaches stack up against each other.

The Numbers Game: AHI Reduction

The Apnea-Hypopnea Index (AHI)—the number of breathing pauses per hour—is the primary measure doctors use to assess sleep apnea severity. When it comes to raw numbers, CPAP maintains a slight edge in AHI reduction when used properly.

Sleep implants, particularly hypoglossal nerve stimulators (HNS), also show impressive results. The landmark STAR trial found that patients using the Inspire system experienced about a 70% reduction in their AHI after one year. Even more encouraging, a five-year follow-up study showed these benefits remained stable over time, with most patients maintaining their improvements.

Did you know?

Comparative studies have found that while CPAP tends to reduce AHI slightly more than HNS (with reductions to around 6.6 events/hour for CPAP versus 8.1 for HNS), both treatments significantly lower AHI, bringing patients from severe sleep apnea into the mild range. These results indicate substantial clinical improvement for both therapies.

In practical terms, this means both treatments can effectively control sleep apnea, though CPAP may achieve slightly lower residual AHI numbers under ideal conditions.

The Real-World Factor: Treatment Adherence

Numbers on paper only matter if patients actually use their treatment. This is where sleep implants shine brightest.

Studies consistently show that about 40-50% of patients prescribed CPAP either abandon it entirely or use it inconsistently within the first year. Even among those who stick with it, many only wear their masks for part of the night.

In contrast, sleep implant users show remarkably high adherence rates. Research indicates that over 90% of patients with hypoglossal nerve stimulators use their devices regularly, typically for the entire night. Since the device is already inside your body, there's no mask to put on or take off—you simply activate it with a remote before bed.

Beyond Numbers: Quality of Life Improvements

Effective treatment isn't just about improving breathing metrics—it's about helping people feel better and live better lives. Both CPAP and sleep implants show significant improvements in daytime functioning and quality of life measures.

Interestingly, some studies suggest that patients with sleep implants report even greater improvements in daytime sleepiness than CPAP users. In one comparative study, HNS patients saw their Epworth Sleepiness Scale scores (a measure of daytime sleepiness) improve by about eight points, compared to four points for CPAP users.

Sleep implant users also report high satisfaction with their treatment. In surveys, many express relief at no longer needing to wear a mask and appreciate the freedom to sleep in any position without worrying about dislodging equipment.

Quality of Life Improvements with Sleep Implants

While CPAP (Continuous Positive Airway Pressure) therapy focuses on keeping the airways open through external pressure, sleep implants work in harmony with your body's natural processes, offering a more integrated approach to treatment. CPAP requires patients to wear a mask and endure the discomfort of continuous airflow, which can be difficult for long-term adherence. In contrast, sleep implants are designed to stimulate the muscles and tissues in the airway, prompting them to stay open during sleep without the need for external equipment. This subtle yet significant difference not only enhances comfort but also leads to improvements in overall sleep quality, particularly for patients who struggle with CPAP adherence or find it disruptive. The body's natural mechanisms are supported rather than overridden, providing a potentially more sustainable and personalized treatment option. As research continues to explore the benefits of sleep implants, early findings suggest they could offer a promising alternative or complement to traditional CPAP therapy, particularly for those with moderate to severe obstructive sleep apnea.

Sleep apnea interferes with the body's ability to move naturally through the different stages of sleep. By preventing the airway from collapsing, sleep implants help restore normal sleep patterns, allowing individuals to reach deep sleep and REM sleep—both of which are crucial for physical recovery and mental well-being.

This restoration of natural sleep patterns has cascading benefits. Patients report waking feeling genuinely refreshed—often for the first time in years. Many describe the sensation as "remembering what normal sleep feels like" after years of fragmented, disrupted rest.

Perhaps the most immediately noticeable benefit for most patients is the dramatic improvement in daytime functioning. Sleep apnea's chronic sleep disruption typically causes debilitating daytime sleepiness, poor concentration, and mental fog.

Studies show that patients using hypoglossal nerve stimulation experience significant improvements in daytime alertness as measured by the Epworth Sleepiness Scale (ESS)—a standard assessment of daytime drowsiness. The STAR trial found that average ESS scores dropped from 11.6 (indicating excessive daytime sleepiness) to 7.0

(within the normal range) after 12 months of therapy.

This cognitive revival extends beyond the workplace. Patients report enjoying books again, having the mental energy for hobbies, and being more present in conversations with loved ones. Many discover they've been operating at reduced capacity for years without realizing it.

Safety Profiles of Sleep Implants

When considering any medical device that lives inside your body, safety naturally becomes a top concern. How safe are sleep implants compared to other sleep apnea treatments? Let's explore what the research tells us about their safety record and what patients should know before considering this option.

Understanding the Risks: Surgical Considerations

Unlike CPAP therapy or oral appliances, hypoglossal nerve stimulators require a surgical procedure to implant. This introduces a unique set of potential risks that don't exist with non-surgical treatments.

The surgical procedure typically involves three small incisions: one under the chin to place the stimulation lead on the hypoglossal nerve, one in the chest for the pulse generator, and one between the ribs for the breathing sensor. It's performed under general anesthesia and usually takes 2-3 hours.

Did you know?

Clinical studies indicate that serious surgical complications from hypoglossal nerve stimulator (HGNS) implantation are rare, making it one of the safer surgical procedures for treating sleep disorders, particularly obstructive sleep apnea. The procedure, which involves implanting a device that stimulates the hypoglossal nerve to prevent airway collapse during sleep, has been associated with a low incidence of complications. Studies have consistently shown that the procedure is well-tolerated by patients, with most reporting significant improvements in sleep quality. Additionally, long-term follow-up data has reinforced the safety profile of hypoglossal nerve stimulation, making it a viable option for patients who are either intolerant of CPAP therapy or are seeking an alternative treatment for more severe cases of obstructive sleep apnea. With its favorable safety and effectiveness, HGNS presents a promising solution for improving sleep apnea management.

Nevertheless, just per the norm and like anything medical in this world, HGNS does pose some risks. Although they are rare, the most common surgical risks include:

- Infection: Occurring in about 1-2% of patients, usually treatable with antibiotics
- Bleeding or hematoma: Typically minor and resolving without intervention
- Temporary tongue weakness: Usually resolves within days or weeks
- Nerve injury: Rare but possible, especially with inexperienced surgeons
- Pain at implant sites: Generally mild and manageable with standard pain medication

Most patients experience mild to moderate discomfort for the first few days after surgery, primarily at the incision sites. This typically resolves within a week and can be managed with over-the-counter pain relievers.

The device isn't activated immediately after surgery. Most physicians wait about a month for complete healing before turning on the stimulation. This allows inflammation to subside and ensures the leads are stable in their final positions.

Long-Term Safety: What the Data Shows

Perhaps the most reassuring aspect of sleep implants is their excellent long-term safety record. The STAR trial, which followed patients for five years after implantation, found no new or unexpected safety concerns emerging over time.

Long-term complications are rare but can include:

- Lead migration: The stimulation lead can occasionally shift position, requiring surgical adjustment (occurs in about 2-3% of patients)
- Device malfunction: Rare electronic failures may require replacement
- Discomfort during stimulation: Usually addressable by adjusting stimulation settings
- Battery depletion: Requires generator replacement after 8-11 years (a minor outpatient procedure)

The risk of serious adverse events is remarkably low. In fact, a 2021 meta-analysis comparing treatment options found that hypoglossal nerve stimulation had fewer serious side effects than surgical options like uvulopalatopharyngoplasty (UPPP) and a comparable safety profile to long-term CPAP use when all health impacts were considered.

Surgical and Post-Surgical Considerations

Getting a sleep implant isn't like picking up a CPAP machine from a medical supply store—it involves surgery and recovery. Understanding what happens before, during, and after the procedure can help patients prepare for this life-changing treatment option.

The Surgical Journey

For a hypoglossal nerve stimulator (the most common sleep implant), surgeons make two or three small incisions: one under the chin to access the hypoglossal nerve, one in the upper chest to place the pulse generator (similar to a pacemaker), and in some cases, a third incision between the ribs to position the breathing sensor.

During the procedure, surgeons carefully identify the specific branch of the hypoglossal nerve that controls tongue protrusion. This precision is crucial—stimulating the wrong nerve branch could actually worsen sleep apnea instead of improving it. Once identified, they gently place a small electrode cuff around this nerve branch.

The procedure is typically performed as outpatient surgery, meaning most patients go home the same day after a brief recovery period and monitoring.

Immediate Post-Operative Care

Waking up with a newly implanted device brings a mix of hope and temporary discomfort. Here's what patients typically experience in those first crucial days:

- Hospital monitoring: Before discharge, patients usually undergo a chest X-ray to confirm proper device placement and rule out complications like pneumothorax (collapsed lung), which is rare but possible when placing the breathing sensor.
- Pain management: Most patients experience mild to moderate pain at the incision sites. "The discomfort is usually manageable with over-the-counter pain relievers," says Dr. Torres. "Some patients might need prescription pain medication for the first few days, but rarely longer than that."
- Antibiotics: A short course of preventive antibiotics is typically prescribed to reduce infection risk.
- Activity restrictions: Patients are advised to avoid strenuous activities and heavy lifting (over ten pounds) for about two weeks to allow proper healing and prevent lead displacement.

The Healing Phase

An important detail that surprises many patients: the device isn't activated immediately. There's typically a waiting period of about one month before the first activation, allowing time for tissue healing, reduction of surgical swelling, and proper integration of the implant with the body. This phase is crucial for ensuring optimal functionality and minimizing complications when the device is eventually turned on.

During this healing phase, patients should follow post-operative care instructions carefully and watch for warning signs that require medical attention:

- Signs of infection: Increasing redness, warmth, swelling, or unusual drainage from incision sites may indicate an infection that requires prompt evaluation. Fever, chills, or a general feeling of illness could also be warning signs.
- Severe or worsening pain: While some discomfort is expected, pain that does not improve with prescribed medication or intensifies over time could signal an underlying issue, such as infection or improper healing.
- Unusual swelling or fluid accumulation: Persistent or asymmetric swelling at the surgical site may suggest fluid buildup (seroma) or hematoma, which might require drainage or medical intervention.
- Numbness, tingling, or weakness: While mild sensory changes near the incision site can be normal, persistent or worsening numbness, tingling, or muscle weakness in the surrounding area may indicate nerve irritation or compression.
- Difficulty swallowing or breathing: Any sensation of tightness, difficulty swallowing, or breathing issues should be evaluated immediately, as post-operative swelling near the airway could cause complications.

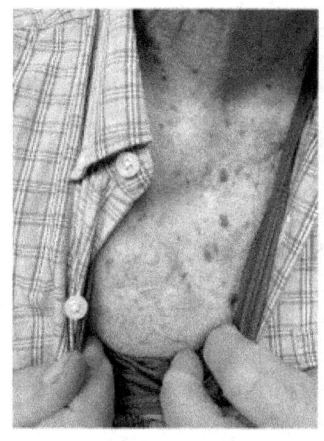
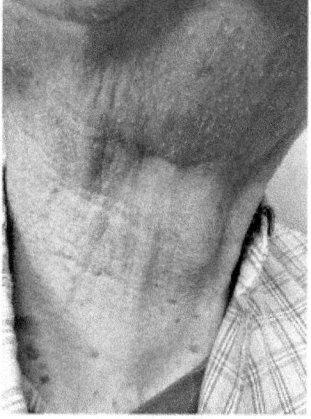

Pictures of incision areas 2-3 months out after surgery — incisions are hardly noticeable

During this period, patients are encouraged to maintain good wound care, avoid excessive physical strain, and follow dietary and activity guidelines provided by their medical team. Attending follow-up appointments is essential to monitor healing progress and address any emerging concerns before device activation.

Once healing is complete, the first activation session marks the next step in the journey, where adjustments are made to ensure the device functions optimally to manage sleep apnea symptoms effectively.

Next-Generation Sleep Implants

Smart Polymer Implants: The Flexible Future

Unlike current devices that use electrical stimulation, smart polymer implants would provide physical support to prevent airway collapse. These innovative materials can change their properties—becoming firmer or more flexible—in response to different stimuli.

Recent proof-of-concept research has shown promising results. In a

2021 study published in SLEEP Advances, researchers demonstrated that smart polymer implants placed in the upper airway could significantly reduce collapsibility during sleep. When combined with weight loss interventions, these implants improved several aspects of sleep apnea, including breathing patterns and arousal thresholds.

Did you know?

According to research by Sideris et al., smart polymer implants could offer a novel solution for sleep apnea by ensuring stable airway support without external devices or continuous electrical stimulation. Scientists at the University of Wollongong are also developing personalized, minimally invasive implants using 3D printing and magnetic fields to maintain airway patency, potentially providing a more tolerable alternative to traditional treatments.

What makes these implants particularly exciting is their potential simplicity. Without batteries or complex electronics, they could last longer and require less maintenance than current neurostimulation devices. Some designs even respond to the body's natural breathing efforts, providing support only when needed.

Miniaturized and Battery-Free Designs

The next generation of sleep implants is getting smaller, smarter, and in some cases, ditching batteries altogether. The Genio system by Nyxoah represents this trend toward miniaturization. Unlike traditional hypoglossal nerve stimulators that require a pulse generator in the chest, the Genio implant is a small chip placed under the chin.

Perhaps the most revolutionary is the move toward battery-free operation. Some emerging implants use external power sources through wireless energy transfer. The patient wears a small external patch or necklace during sleep that wirelessly powers the implant. This approach eliminates the need for battery replacement surgery and allows for even smaller implant designs.

Artificial Intelligence and Adaptive Stimulation

Current sleep implants deliver relatively standardized stimulation based on breathing patterns. The next generation of these devices, however, is expected to integrate artificial intelligence (AI) to provide personalized, adaptive therapy that meets each patient's unique needs. This innovation promises to enhance both the effectiveness and comfort of sleep apnea treatment.

AI-enhanced implants could potentially:

Adapt to changing needs: The device would automatically adjust therapy as your condition evolves, ensuring continuous optimization over time.

Predict apnea events: By identifying patterns that precede breathing pauses, the implant could intervene proactively, preventing disruptions before they occur.

Optimize for comfort: AI could fine-tune the balance between effective therapy and minimal sensation, improving comfort without compromising treatment.

Provide detailed sleep insights: The implant would gather and analyze sleep data, offering valuable insights that could help refine therapy and monitor progress.

Conclusion and Transition

Throughout this chapter, we've taken a fascinating journey into the world of sleep implants—a revolutionary approach that's changing how we treat sleep apnea. Let's pull together the key insights we've discovered about these remarkable devices and what they mean for patients seeking alternatives to CPAP therapy.

The evidence is compelling: sleep implants work. Studies consistently show that hypoglossal nerve stimulation (HNS) devices can reduce sleep apnea events by 60-70% in appropriate candidates. The landmark STAR trial demonstrated that most patients achieved significant improvements, with their Apnea-Hypopnea Index (AHI) dropping from severe levels to the mild range.

Looking forward to Chapter 3, we move beyond the science and technology to explore what happens once a patient says "yes" to a sleep implant. From surgery prep and early recovery to activation, adjustment, and long-term impact, you'll witness the full patient journey unfold. Through personal stories and clinical insights, we'll explore the emotional, physical, and practical realities of living with a sleep implant—and what it truly takes to turn treatment into transformation.

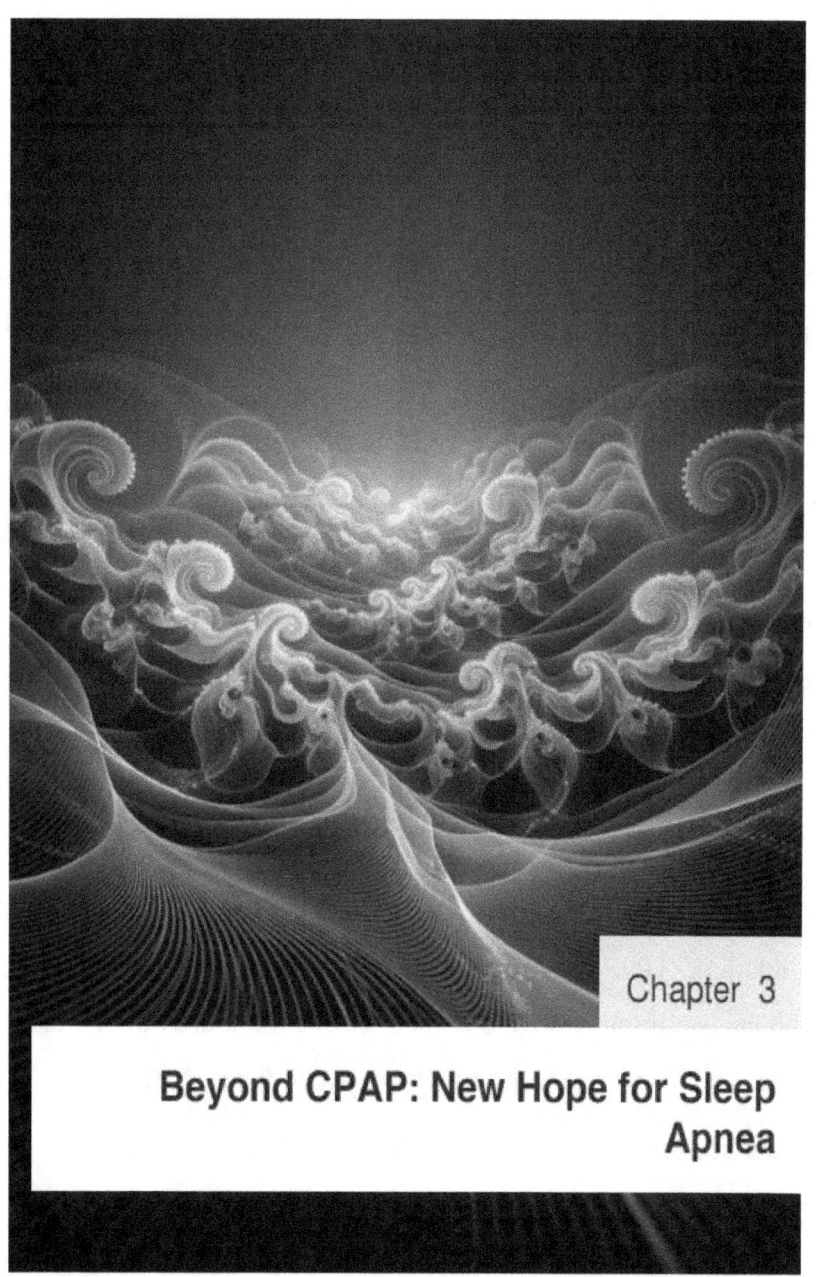

Chapter 3

Beyond CPAP: New Hope for Sleep Apnea

Chapter 3:
Types of Sleep Implants and Their Application

Exploring the Implant Landscape

So, you've learned that sleep apnea can quietly wreak havoc on your health—and that sleep implants are emerging as powerful alternatives to the dreaded CPAP machine. But here's the question we're tackling now: What exactly are these implants, and who are they for?

It's not a one-size-fits-all solution. In fact, there's an entire ecosystem of sleep implants designed to meet different needs—each with its own mechanics, benefits, and ideal candidate. Think of it like choosing the right tool for the job: tongue-based obstruction? There's a device for that. Central sleep apnea? That calls for something else entirely. No teeth to anchor an oral appliance? There's a workaround for that, too.

In this chapter, we'll dive into the world of sleep implants as they exist today—starting with the most established approach: hypoglossal nerve stimulation (HNS). You'll learn how doctors determine whether someone is eligible, how the implant works night after night, and what kind of results patients are actually seeing in the real world.

But we won't stop there. We'll explore new frontiers, too—from dental innovations to combination therapies that take sleep treatment to the next level. Because when it comes to breathing better at night, no option should be off the table.

Patient Eligibility for HNS

Indeed, determining who's a good candidate for HNS involves a careful screening process. Unlike CPAP therapy, which can be prescribed for almost any sleep apnea patient, HNS works best for specific types of patients with particular characteristics. Unlike CPAP therapy, which can be prescribed to a broad range of patients, HNS is most effective for individuals with moderate to severe obstructive sleep apnea who have not found success with CPAP or other less invasive treatments. The goal of this careful selection process is to identify candidates who are most likely to benefit from the procedure, maximizing the potential for successful outcomes and improved sleep quality. This careful selection process helps ensure the best possible outcomes for those who undergo the procedure.

Think of HNS eligibility as finding a "Goldilocks zone" where everything is just right. The ideal candidate falls within specific parameters for several key factors:

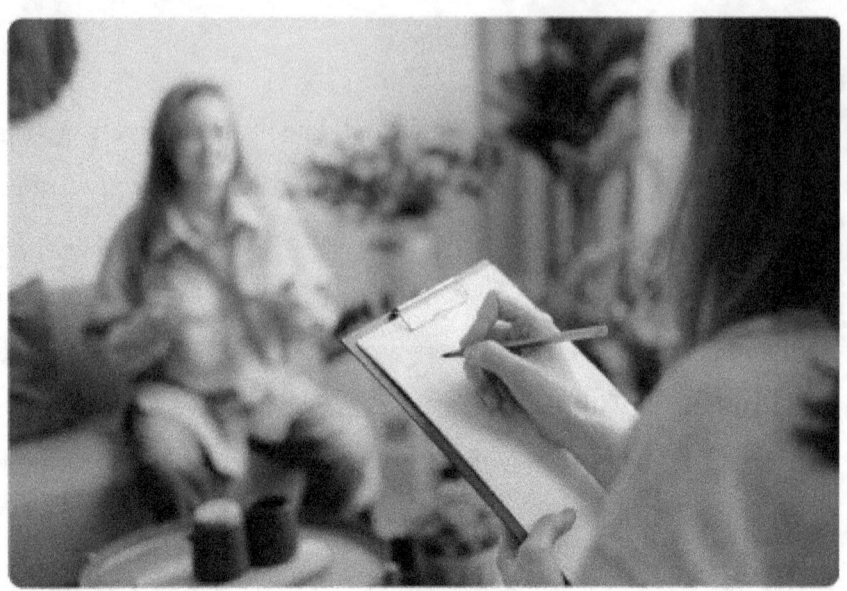

Consultation before further interventions. Photo credit: Pexels.

- Sleep Apnea Severity: Patients need to have moderate to severe obstructive sleep apnea, typically with an apnea-hypopnea index (AHI) between 15 and 65 events per hour. This means your breathing stops or becomes shallow between 15 and 65 times each hour during sleep. If your sleep apnea is too mild (below 15), the benefits may not outweigh the risks of surgery. If it's extremely severe (above 65), HNS might not be powerful enough to overcome such significant airway collapse.
- Body Weight: Most guidelines require patients to have a body mass index (BMI) below 35. Some centers may accept patients with slightly higher BMIs on a case-by-case basis. This requirement exists because excess weight, especially around the neck, can create too much pressure for nerve stimulation to

overcome. Sandra was initially concerned about this requirement: "I was right at the borderline with a BMI of 34. My doctor explained that losing even a small amount of weight would improve my chances of success with the device."

- CPAP Experience: Patients must have tried and been unable to use or benefit from CPAP therapy. This could mean you're unable to tolerate the mask, experience claustrophobia, travel frequently, or simply can't achieve good results despite consistent use. Insurance typically requires documented CPAP failure before approving HNS.

Did you know?

A 2022 study in the *Journal of Clinical Sleep Medicine* found that approximately 50-60% of sleep apnea patients struggle with CPAP adherence, making alternative treatments like HNS particularly valuable. However, of those patients, only about 20-30% meet all the eligibility criteria for HNS therapy, highlighting the importance of careful patient selection.

Looking Inside: The Critical Airway Assessment

Perhaps the most unique aspect of hypoglossal nerve stimulation (HNS) eligibility is the thorough evaluation of airway anatomy. Not all types of airway collapse respond equally well to this therapy, making precise assessment crucial in determining whether a patient will benefit from the implant. To identify suitable candidates, physicians rely on a specialized diagnostic procedure known as drug-induced sleep endoscopy (DISE).

What Happens During a DISE Procedure?

DISE is a minimally invasive examination performed in a controlled environment, typically in an operating room or sleep lab. During the procedure, the patient is given a sedative to induce a sleep-like state that closely mimics natural sleep patterns. A thin, flexible endoscope is then inserted through the nose and advanced into the airway, allowing the physician to directly observe how the airway behaves when relaxed.

Key Observations in DISE

As the endoscope provides real-time visualization, the physician carefully evaluates several factors:

- Site of Airway Collapse: The primary goal of DISE is to identify the exact location where the obstruction occurs. HNS is most effective for patients whose airway obstruction is concentrated at the base of the tongue. If the primary collapse occurs at the soft palate or in multiple areas simultaneously, alternative treatment approaches may be more appropriate.
- Pattern of Collapse: Not all airway blockages behave the same way. Physicians classify collapse patterns into different categories. HNS is most successful when the obstruction is an anteroposterior collapse (where the tongue moves backward into the airway). However, if a patient exhibits "concentric collapse" at the soft palate—where the airway closes in a

circular manner—HNS is generally less effective, and other interventions may be recommended.

- Severity and Stability of Collapse: The degree of obstruction and its consistency throughout different sleep stages are also assessed. Some patients may have intermittent airway closure, while others experience more severe and sustained obstruction.

Why DISE Matters for HNS Success

DISE plays a crucial role in ensuring the best possible outcomes for HNS patients. By precisely mapping how the airway collapses, doctors can determine whether stimulation of the hypoglossal nerve will provide meaningful relief. If a patient's airway anatomy is favorable, the likelihood of successful treatment increases significantly.

For individuals who do not meet the criteria for HNS due to their specific airway collapse pattern, alternative treatment options—such as CPAP therapy, positional therapy, or upper airway surgery—may be explored. Ultimately, DISE serves as a critical step in personalizing sleep apnea treatment, ensuring that patients receive the most effective and appropriate intervention for their condition.

Clinical Evidence of HNS

The landmark Stimulation Therapy for Apnea Reduction (STAR) trial stands as the cornerstone of evidence supporting HNS therapy. This groundbreaking study tracked patients with moderate-to-severe sleep apnea who couldn't use or benefit from CPAP therapy.

The results were eye-opening: After 12 months of using the Inspire system, participants experienced a 68% reduction in their apnea-hypopnea index (AHI)—the number of breathing pauses or shallow breaths per hour. Their AHI dropped from an average of 29.3 events per hour to just 9.0 events per hour. For context, an AHI below 15 is considered only mild sleep apnea, so many patients improved from severe or moderate to mild levels.

Even more impressively, about two-thirds of participants achieved what researchers call "treatment success"—their AHI decreased by at least 50% and fell below 20 events per hour. These benefits weren't just short-term wins; follow-up studies showed they persisted at three and five years after implantation.

Comparing Apples to Apples: HNS vs. CPAP

How does HNS stack up against CPAP therapy? This is tricky to answer directly since most HNS studies focus on patients who couldn't use CPAP. However, some comparative data exists.

When comparing the results of patients who successfully use either therapy, CPAP and HNS show similar improvements in key metrics like AHI reduction and daytime sleepiness. The critical difference lies in usage patterns. CPAP is highly effective—when people use it. However, studies show that 30-50% of patients prescribed CPAP either abandon it entirely or use it inconsistently.

In contrast, HNS shows remarkable adherence and consistent results, offering a reliable alternative for those who struggle with CPAP.

Future Directions in HNS Technology

Current HNS devices typically have batteries that last 8–10 years before requiring surgical replacement. While this is already impressive compared to many medical devices, researchers are working on two parallel paths to improve this aspect of the technology.

First, next-generation batteries aim to extend device longevity to 15+ years, significantly reducing the need for replacement surgeries. Second, and perhaps more revolutionary, are wirelessly rechargeable systems that would eliminate replacement surgeries altogether.

Perhaps the most exciting advancement is the development of "smart" HNS systems that can adapt to individual patients' needs in real time. Current devices deliver consistent stimulation based on settings programmed during clinical visits. Future devices aim to be much more responsive and personalized.

These advanced systems will incorporate artificial intelligence to learn a patient's unique breathing patterns and adjust stimulation accordingly. For example, if a patient's apnea worsens in certain sleep positions or during REM sleep, the device would automatically increase stimulation during those times.

Role of Dental Implants in OSA

The connection between dental health and sleep breathing disorders is becoming increasingly recognized in sleep medicine. For patients with obstructive sleep apnea (OSA) who struggle with traditional treatments like CPAP or even newer options like hypoglossal nerve stimulation (HNS), dental implants are emerging as a promising alternative—or complementary—approach.

Dental implants serve as artificial tooth roots, typically made of titanium, that are surgically placed into the jawbone. While they're primarily used to replace missing teeth, their role in sleep apnea treatment is both innovative and multifaceted. In particular, they allow for the successful use of mandibular advancement devices (MADs) in patients who are fully or partially edentulous (missing some or all of their teeth).

Traditionally, MADs work by anchoring to natural teeth and repositioning the lower jaw forward during sleep. This forward shift reduces airway obstruction by preventing the tongue and soft tissues from collapsing backward. However, for patients without sufficient teeth, especially those who are completely edentulous, anchoring these devices has been a major limitation—until now.

By strategically placing dental implants in the upper or lower jaw, clinicians can create a stable foundation to retain custom sleep apnea appliances. These implant-supported oral appliances come in various designs:

- Bar-retained appliances: A rigid bar is secured to multiple implants (usually four or more), and the oral appliance snaps onto the bar with precision clip attachments. This system ensures that the appliance stays firmly in place throughout the night, even without natural teeth.

- Locator-retained appliances: These use individual implant "stud" attachments that allow for direct snap-on mechanisms. Patients may wear a removable oral appliance that clicks into place on top of the implants, offering reliable retention without needing upper or lower dentures during sleep.
- Overdenture-integrated devices: In some cases, MADs are designed to fit over existing implant-supported dentures, combining daily denture functionality with nighttime airway support.

Studies have shown that these implant-supported MADs can significantly reduce the apnea-hypopnea index (AHI) in edentulous patients—sometimes bringing it down from moderate or severe to mild or even normal levels. In one landmark pilot study, patients treated with mandibular implants and a bar-retained advancement appliance experienced marked improvements in oxygen levels, sleep quality, and daytime alertness.

For patients who cannot tolerate CPAP and have no other non-surgical options, dental implants open the door to effective, long-term therapy. They are especially useful in combination therapy, allowing for enhanced stability when paired with other interventions such as positional therapy or even low-pressure CPAP use.

While implant-supported appliances require more time and investment upfront, they offer a high level of patient satisfaction, comfort, and compliance. They've transformed what was once a contraindicated population—edentulous patients—into active candidates for oral appliance therapy.

As dental sleep medicine continues to evolve, implant-supported appliances are expected to play a growing role—bridging the gap between oral prosthetics and respiratory care and offering new hope to patients who've long been underserved.

Combination Therapy Options

The field of sleep medicine increasingly recognizes that sleep apnea is a complex condition that often benefits from multi-modal treatment. Implant therapies like hypoglossal nerve stimulation can work even better when paired with other interventions. This combined approach addresses sleep apnea from multiple angles, often yielding results greater than the sum of their parts.

CPAP and Implant Therapy: Unexpected Partners

At first glance, combining CPAP with an implant might seem counterintuitive. After all, many patients pursue implants specifically to avoid CPAP. However, this combination can be remarkably effective in certain scenarios.

For patients with severe sleep apnea (AHI > 30), an implant alone might not provide complete resolution. By adding CPAP at a lower, more comfortable pressure setting, patients can experience better results while avoiding the discomfort of high-pressure CPAP.

Did you know?

A 2023 case report published in *The Journal of Clinical Sleep Medicine* described a successful use of combination therapy with hypoglossal nerve stimulation (HNS) and CPAP in a patient with severe obstructive sleep apnea (OSA) who had previously struggled with CPAP adherence. The patient experienced a significant reduction in apnea events, with a 56% decrease in AHI and marked improvements in sleep quality and mask retention.

Positional Therapy: A Simple but Powerful Addition

Many sleep apnea patients experience worse symptoms when sleeping on their backs (supine position). In this position, gravity increases the likelihood of airway collapse, exacerbating breathing disruptions. For individuals whose sleep apnea is primarily position-dependent, integrating positional therapy into their treatment plan can provide significant benefits, particularly when used alongside implant therapy.

Positional therapy aims to encourage side sleeping, which can help maintain better airway patency throughout the night. A variety of methods and devices can support this approach:

- Simple behavioral techniques: Some patients find success with low-tech solutions, such as sewing a tennis ball into the back of a sleep shirt or using a specially designed pillow to discourage back sleeping. While inexpensive and straightforward, these methods require consistency and adaptation over time.
- Advanced positional therapy devices: More sophisticated electronic positioners offer an effective and user-friendly

alternative. These devices detect when a person rolls onto their back and provide gentle vibrations to encourage repositioning without fully waking the sleeper. Some models integrate with sleep-tracking apps, offering insights into sleep patterns and compliance.

- Adjustable beds and body positioning aids: Elevating the head of the bed or using body-positioning pillows can also reduce the severity of positional sleep apnea by preventing the airway from fully collapsing.

When combined with implant therapy, positional therapy can enhance treatment effectiveness, leading to greater symptom relief and improved sleep quality. Patients who struggle with residual apnea events despite implant activation may find that addressing body position provides an additional layer of control over their condition.

Exercise: Beyond Just Weight Loss

Regular physical activity offers benefits for sleep apnea patients that extend well beyond weight management. While maintaining a healthy weight can reduce the severity of obstructive sleep apnea (OSA) by decreasing fat deposits around the airway, exercise contributes to improved sleep health in several additional ways. Engaging in consistent physical activity enhances overall sleep architecture, reduces systemic inflammation, and strengthens the muscles that help maintain airway patency.

Studies suggest that moderate to vigorous exercise can lead to deeper, more restorative sleep, even in individuals who do not experience significant weight loss. Regular movement helps regulate the autonomic nervous system, lowering sympathetic activity (which is often elevated in sleep apnea patients) and reducing the frequency of nighttime awakenings. Additionally, exercise has been shown to improve daytime energy levels, reduce symptoms of excessive daytime sleepiness, and enhance overall cardiovascular health—critical factors for individuals managing sleep apnea.

Targeted Upper Airway Exercises

In addition to general aerobic and resistance training, exercises specifically designed to strengthen the upper airway muscles can be particularly beneficial. These exercises help improve airway stability by increasing muscle tone and reducing airway collapsibility during sleep. Among the most effective methods are:

- Oropharyngeal exercises (myofunctional therapy): These involve targeted movements for the tongue, soft palate, and throat muscles. Studies indicate that consistent practice of these exercises can reduce apnea severity by improving airway muscle tone.
- Singing and vocal training: Certain vocal exercises help strengthen the muscles of the soft palate and throat, improving airway control. Some research suggests that structured singing programs can reduce snoring and mild-to-moderate OSA symptoms.

- Playing wind instruments: Instruments such as the didgeridoo have been studied for their role in strengthening the airway muscles. The circular breathing technique required for these instruments has been associated with a reduction in apnea events.
- Jaw and tongue exercises: Strengthening the tongue and improving its positioning can prevent it from falling backward and obstructing the airway. Simple exercises, such as tongue presses against the roof of the mouth and resistance exercises with a spoon or rubber band, can be incorporated into a daily routine.

When these targeted exercises are performed consistently alongside implant therapy, they can enhance the tone of the very muscles the implant stimulates during sleep. This complementary approach may lead to more stable breathing patterns and better long-term outcomes for sleep apnea patients.

Sleep Positioning and Bedroom Environment

The way you sleep at night isn't just a matter of comfort—it can play a big role in how well your sleep apnea implant performs. For many patients, especially those using hypoglossal nerve stimulation (HNS) devices, sleep position can either support or work against the therapy. Back-sleeping, for example, allows gravity to pull the tongue and soft tissues backward, which can obstruct the airway even when the implant is doing its job. Side-sleeping, on the other hand, is often more implant-friendly and can help keep your airway open more effectively.

Many patients find that simply switching to side sleeping significantly improves their sleep quality. If you're not used to sleeping this way, small adjustments can help—like hugging a body pillow, placing a cushion behind your back to prevent rolling over or using a wedge pillow to keep your head and torso slightly elevated. These changes can support both comfort and airway alignment throughout the night.

In addition to sleep position, your bedroom environment has a major impact on the quality of your rest. A calm, cool, and quiet space sets the stage for deeper, uninterrupted sleep, which gives your implant the best chance to work effectively. Consider these key environmental tips:

- Temperature control: Keeping your bedroom cool—ideally around 65–68°F (18–20°C)—helps your body settle into deeper sleep stages.
- Light management: Use blackout curtains or an eye mask to reduce light exposure, especially early in the morning or from outside sources.
- Noise reduction: Use white noise machines, fans, or soft earplugs to block disruptive sounds and create a peaceful sleep setting.
- Consistent sleep schedule: Going to bed and waking up at the same times daily helps regulate your body's natural rhythm and reinforces your implant's nightly routine.

By making small changes to how—and where—you sleep, you can enhance both the comfort and the effectiveness of your sleep apnea treatment. When your environment and body are aligned, your implant can do its job with fewer obstacles, helping you breathe easier and wake up feeling truly refreshed.

Conclusion and Transition

As we've explored throughout this chapter, sleep implants represent a revolutionary approach to treating obstructive sleep apnea. From the established Inspire hypoglossal nerve stimulation system to emerging dental implant technologies, these innovations offer hope to countless patients who struggle with traditional CPAP therapy.

Perhaps the most exciting trend on the horizon is the move toward truly personalized sleep medicine. This personalization is already beginning with current technologies. The combination therapy approaches we've discussed—pairing implants with oral appliances, lifestyle changes, or modified CPAP—represent early steps toward customized treatment plans. But future advancements will take this concept much further.

Looking forward to Chapter 4, we will shift from the technology itself to the human experience behind it. You'll follow real patients through every stage of the sleep implant journey—from the anticipation before surgery to the challenges of recovery, the excitement of activation, and the transformation that follows. This next chapter will give you a behind-the-scenes look at what it truly means to live with a sleep implant and how collaborative care, lifestyle changes, and persistence all come together to create a lasting impact.

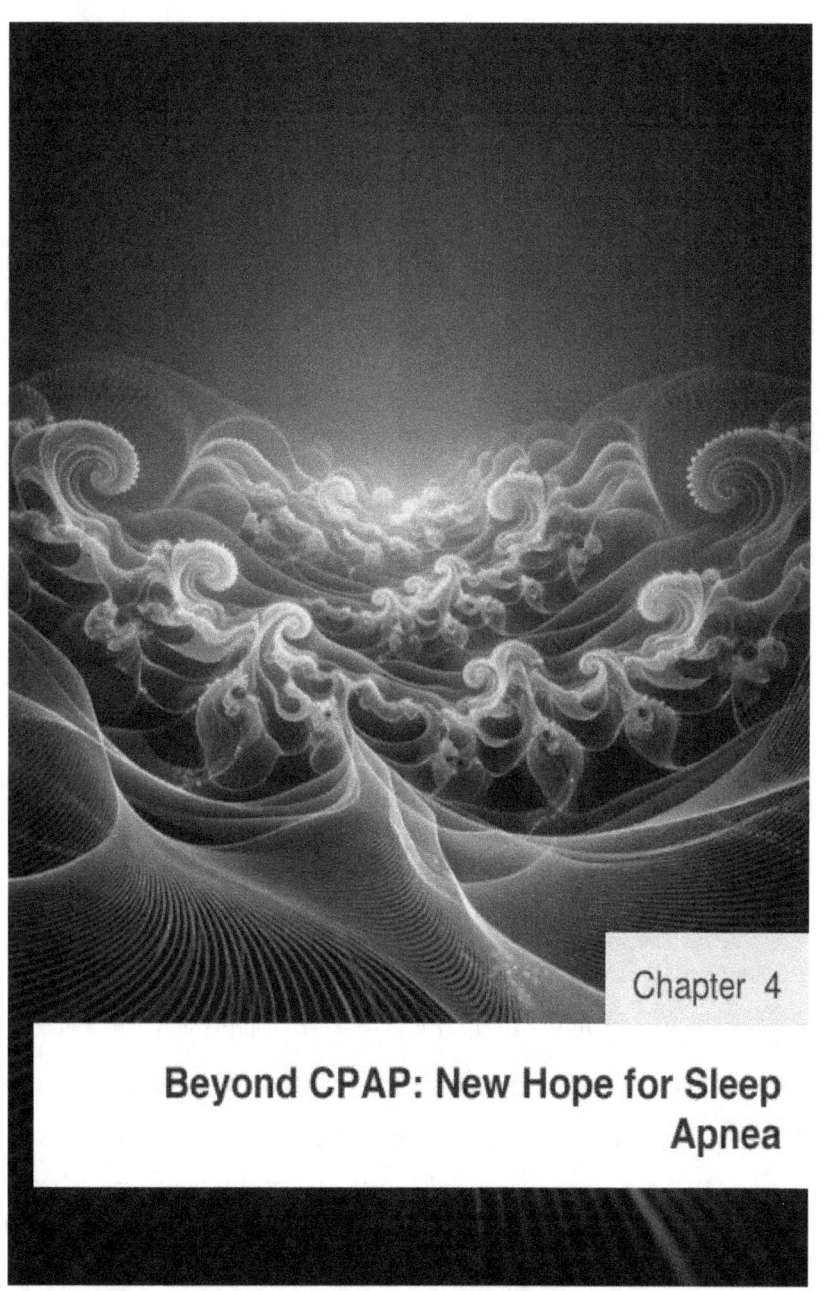

Chapter 4

Beyond CPAP: New Hope for Sleep Apnea

Chapter 4:

The Patient Journey with Sleep Implants

The Road to Restorative Sleep

Receiving a sleep implant isn't just about signing up for surgery—it's a journey, a partnership, and a transformation. For many patients, it begins with frustration: years of battling CPAP machines, struggling to stay awake during the day, and searching for answers that finally lead to the possibility of something different. But what happens after that moment of hope?

This chapter is all about what comes next: the patient journey. From the first surgical consultation to the night you finally sleep soundly without interruptions, getting a sleep implant is a process shaped by teamwork, preparation, and ongoing adjustment.

Behind every successful implant is a well-coordinated care team. It's not just one doctor calling the shots—it's a collaboration between your sleep specialist, ENT surgeon, anesthesiologist, primary care provider, and others. Each plays a distinct role in shaping your care plan. Together, they ensure your anatomy, health history, and treatment goals align with the implant's capabilities. Often, your case may be discussed in a team meeting or case conference to fine-tune the strategy—because in sleep medicine, personalized care is everything.

Once you've been approved, the real adventure begins. Surgery is just one milestone. Recovery, adjustment, activation, titration—it's all part of learning to live with this small but powerful device inside you. And as we'll see in the stories ahead, that process comes with both challenges and life-changing rewards.

Let's walk through what this journey really looks like—from recovery hurdles and first-night nerves to full-on life transformation.

Patient Testimonials: Overcoming Initial Challenges

Maria was thrilled when she finally qualified for her sleep implant. After years of struggling with her CPAP mask—fighting with tangled tubing, dealing with dry sinuses, and waking up to find she'd removed the mask in her sleep—she was ready for something different. But the day after her implant surgery, she called her doctor in a panic.

"I feel this weird tugging sensation when I swallow, and there's some soreness where they put in the device," she explained. "Is this normal? Did something go wrong?"

Maria's experience is common among new sleep implant recipients. While these devices offer life-changing benefits for many patients, the journey isn't without its bumps. Let's explore the real-world challenges that patients face in those crucial first weeks and months—and how they overcome them.

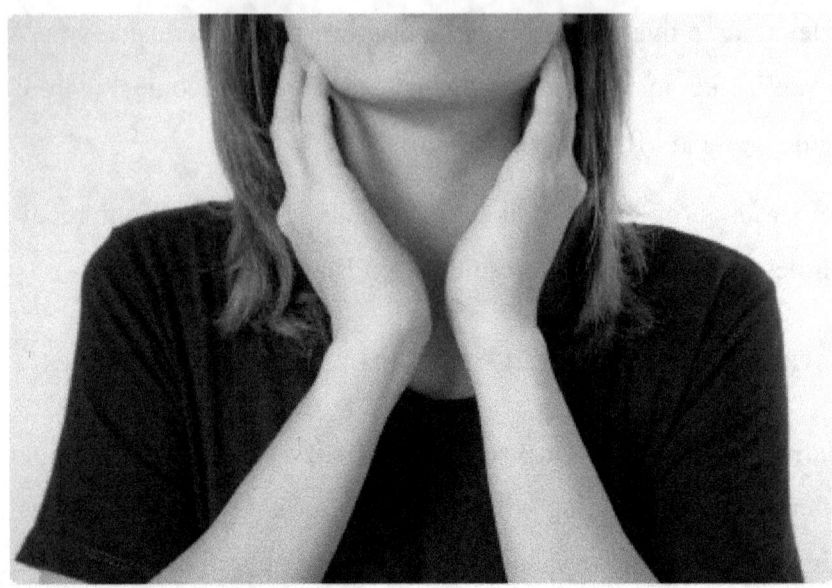

Neck can be a common area of post-surgical discomfort. Photo credit: Pexels

The First Few Days: Surgical Recovery Hurdles

The immediate post-surgical period brings its own set of challenges. For Tom, a 58-year-old former CPAP user, the first week after his hypoglossal nerve stimulator implantation tested his resolve.

- Incision site pain: Most patients report mild to moderate discomfort at the surgical sites, particularly the chest pocket where the pulse generator is implanted.
- Swallowing discomfort: The sensing lead placed between the rib muscles can cause a temporary sensation of "tugging" when swallowing.
- Sleep position limitations: Patients often need to avoid sleeping on the side where the device is implanted for several weeks.

- Voice changes: Some patients notice temporary hoarseness or voice fatigue.

For Maria, her doctor's reassurance made all the difference. "He told me these sensations were completely normal and would fade as healing progressed," she says. "Just knowing that helped me relax and trust the process."

The Waiting Game: Activation Anticipation

Unlike CPAP, which patients begin using immediately, most sleep implants aren't activated right away. This waiting period—typically 4-6 weeks to allow for healing—can test patients' patience.

"Those weeks of waiting were harder than I expected," admits John, a 45-year-old who received an Inspire implant after a decade of unsuccessful CPAP use. "I was still having sleep apnea symptoms but couldn't use my old CPAP because I'd already given it away. I kept reminding myself it was temporary, but some nights were rough."

- Positional therapy: Using specialized pillows to maintain side-sleeping and avoid lying flat on their back
- Sleep hygiene practices: Maintaining consistent sleep schedules and bedtime routines
- Temporary oral appliances: Some doctors prescribe dental devices as a bridge during the healing phase

Finding the Sweet Spot: Titration Challenges

When activation day finally arrives, patients eagerly anticipate the benefits of their sleep implant. However, the initial titration process can be challenging as the device settings are adjusted to suit individual needs. Patients often experience a period of adjustment as they find the optimal settings for their implant.

Overall, despite the initial hurdles, many patients find that the long-term benefits of sleep implants far outweigh the initial challenges, leading to improved sleep quality and overall well-being.

Narrative: Life after Sleep Implants

When Michael first received his sleep implant, he wasn't sure what to expect. After years of wrestling with his CPAP mask and waking up exhausted despite using it, he had taken the leap to try something new. Now, eighteen months later, he sits across from me in a coffee shop, energetically describing how his life has transformed.

"The first few weeks were an adjustment," he admits with a smile. "But now? I feel like I've gotten my life back. I never realized how much my sleep apnea was stealing from me until I finally experienced what good sleep actually feels like."

The Transformation Timeline

Life with a sleep implant doesn't change overnight. For most patients, improvements follow a fairly predictable timeline once they've moved past the initial recovery and adjustment period:

- 1-3 months: Most patients notice their first significant improvements in sleep quality. Morning headaches often disappear, and many report feeling more refreshed upon waking.
- 3-6 months: Energy levels typically show marked improvement. Patients find they no longer need afternoon naps and can make it through the day without feeling exhausted.
- 6-12 months: This is when many patients report the most dramatic quality of life improvements, including better mood, improved concentration, and enhanced performance at work.
- Beyond 12 months: Long-term health benefits become more apparent, including improved blood pressure readings and better management of conditions like diabetes.

For Jennifer, a 48-year-old teacher who received her implant two years ago, the changes were gradual but profound. "I didn't wake up the day after activation feeling like a new person," she explains. "But looking back now, the difference between my life then and my life now is night and day. I used to struggle to stay awake during afternoon meetings. Now I'm the one suggesting after-work activities."

Did you know?

Research suggests that sleep implants offer significantly better long-term adherence compared to CPAP therapy, as they eliminate common discomforts like masks, hoses, and noise. While CPAP adherence remains a challenge, patient testimonials indicate that implant users experience greater satisfaction and continued device usage over time. Future studies will help quantify these differences in adherence more precisely.

Sleep Quality: The Foundation of Everything

The most immediate and noticeable change for most patients is improved sleep quality. Without the constant interruptions caused by breathing pauses, sleep becomes more continuous and restorative.

"I used to wake up 30-40 times each night without even realizing it," says David, a 56-year-old accountant who received his implant three years ago. "My sleep study showed I was barely getting any deep sleep or REM sleep. Now, I dream almost every night, which my doctor says is a good sign that I'm getting the deep sleep my body needs."

This improvement in sleep architecture—the natural progression through different sleep stages—has cascading benefits. Patients report:

- Fewer awakenings during the night
- Reduced snoring, often to the delight of sleep partners
- Less dry mouth and throat irritation in the morning
- More vivid dreams, indicating better REM sleep
- Feeling truly refreshed upon waking, often for the first time in years

Daytime Energy: Reclaiming Waking Hours

As sleep quality improves, the fog of daytime fatigue begins to lift. This transformation in energy levels affects virtually every aspect of patients' lives.

"I feel like I have a whole new lease on life," describes one patient, echoing the sentiments of many who have undergone the procedure. With newfound energy, patients often find themselves more engaged in activities they once avoided, leading to a more fulfilling daily life.

Integrating Sleep Implants into Daily Life

When Elena received her sleep implant last year, she thought the surgery would be the hardest part of her journey. "I was so focused on getting through the procedure that I didn't really think about what would come next," she laughs. "Nobody told me there's a whole adjustment period where you're learning to live with this new device inside you. It's like getting a new roommate—one that lives in your body!"

Living with a sleep implant is dramatically different from using a CPAP machine. There's no mask to put on, no hose to untangle, and no machine noise—but that doesn't mean there aren't adjustments to make and habits to develop. Let's explore what daily life actually looks like when you have a device working inside you while you sleep.

The Nightly Ritual: Activating Your Silent Partner

For most sleep implant users, bedtime includes a simple but important step: turning on their device. Mark, who received his hypoglossal nerve stimulator two years ago, describes his routine: "Every night before bed, I grab my small remote control from my nightstand. I press the power button and feel a slight tingling sensation under my tongue that tells me it's working, and that's it. The device is programmed to start stimulation 30 minutes after I turn it on, giving me time to fall asleep before it begins."

This activation process is typically quick and straightforward:

- Power up: Using a small remote control (about the size of a TV remote), you activate the device before getting into bed.

- Delay period: Most devices are programmed with a 30-minute delay before stimulation begins, though this can be adjusted based on how quickly you typically fall asleep.
- Auto-operation: Once activated, the device monitors your breathing patterns and provides stimulation automatically throughout the night.
- Morning deactivation: When you wake up, you simply turn off the device using the same remote.

Adjusting to the Sensations

One of the biggest adjustments for new implant users is getting used to the physical sensations the device creates. Unlike CPAP, which you can feel and hear externally, a sleep implant creates internal sensations that can feel strange at first.

"When my device activates, I feel a gentle tugging sensation under my tongue," explains Sophia, who has had her implant for three years. "At first, it was distracting—I'd focus on it and wonder if it was working right. But after a few weeks, it became so normal that I barely notice it anymore. It's like how you stop noticing the feeling of wearing a watch after a while."

Common sensations patients report include:

- A mild tingling or pulsing under the tongue
- A gentle, rhythmic movement of the tongue
- A slight feeling of muscle contraction in the throat

For most patients, these sensations become background noise within a few weeks as the brain adapts to them. However, the adjustment period varies from person to person.

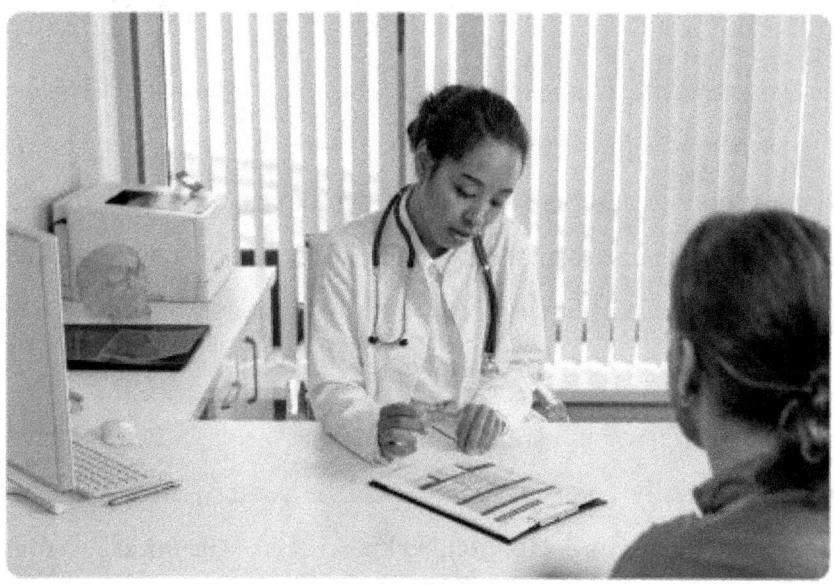

Discussion with a Sleep Specialist. Photo credit: Pexels.

Fine-Tuning for Comfort and Effectiveness

Unlike a one-size-fits-all approach, sleep implants require personalization to work optimally. This means regular follow-up appointments, especially in the first year, to adjust settings based on your comfort and response.

"I've had my settings adjusted three times," says Robert, 18 months after his implantation. "Each adjustment made the device more comfortable and effective for me." Regular check-ins with a specialist ensure the device is finely tuned to meet individual needs, enhancing both comfort and sleep quality.

Optimizing Health and Well-Being Post-Implants

When James received his sleep implant last year, he thought the hardest part was behind him. The surgery had gone well, the device was working properly, and his sleep apnea symptoms were finally under control. But three months later, he found himself in his doctor's office again—not because of any problem with the implant, but because he wasn't feeling as good as he expected.

"I'm sleeping better, but I still feel tired during the day," he explained. "And I've actually gained weight since the surgery, which doesn't make sense to me." His doctor nodded knowingly. "The implant is only one piece of the puzzle," she explained. "Now we need to focus on your overall health to get the full benefits."

Beyond the Device: Creating a Holistic Recovery Plan

A sleep implant can dramatically improve your breathing during sleep, but it works best when supported by healthy lifestyle choices. Think of your implant as the foundation of a house—essential, but not the entire structure. To build your best health, you'll need to add several important elements.

Dr. Elena Martinez, a sleep specialist who works with implant patients, explains: "Many patients think the implant is a magic solution that will fix everything. It's an amazing technology, but it works best when patients take an active role in their overall health. We see the best outcomes in those who address all aspects of their well-being."

Nutrition: Fueling Your Recovery and Beyond

What you eat plays a crucial role in your post-implant journey. While you'll need to follow specific dietary guidelines immediately after surgery (typically soft foods for a week or two), your long-term nutrition strategy can significantly impact your results.

Here's what nutrition experts recommend for sleep implant patients:

- Anti-inflammatory foods: Colorful fruits and vegetables, fatty fish, nuts, and olive oil can help reduce inflammation and support healing.
- Protein-rich options: Adequate protein supports tissue repair and immune function during recovery.

- Weight management: If you're carrying extra weight, gradual weight loss can enhance your implant's effectiveness. Even a 10% reduction in body weight can significantly improve sleep apnea severity.
- Timing matters: Try to finish eating at least three hours before bedtime to prevent reflux and discomfort that might interfere with your sleep.

James found that making gradual changes to his diet made a noticeable difference. "I started eating more vegetables and lean proteins and cut back on processed foods. Within a month, I had more energy during the day, and my implant seemed to work even better."

Movement: Finding Your Exercise Sweet Spot

Physical activity is another crucial element of post-implant wellness. Regular exercise can improve sleep quality, boost energy levels, support weight management, and reduce stress—all factors that complement your implant therapy.

The key is finding activities you enjoy and can sustain. For Lisa, who received her implant two years ago, walking made all the difference. "I started with just ten minutes a day, and now I'm up to 45 minutes most days. I sleep more deeply, and my mood is so much better."

Exercise recommendations for sleep implant patients include:

- Start gradually: Begin with light activities like walking, swimming, or gentle yoga, especially in the first few months after surgery.
- Aim for consistency: Regular, moderate exercise is better than occasional intense workouts.

Conclusion and Transition

The patient journey with sleep implants is a comprehensive process that goes beyond simply receiving a device. From the importance of accurate diagnosis and utilizing validated screening tools to selecting the right testing method, every step in the journey plays a crucial role in ensuring the most effective treatment. As we've seen through the patient experiences shared in this chapter, the transition from traditional CPAP therapy to sleep implants can be life-changing, offering patients improved sleep quality, energy levels, and overall well-being. However, it's clear that successful outcomes depend on careful preoperative planning, personalized care, and ongoing lifestyle adjustments.

Looking forward to Chapter 5, we will explore the critical relationship between metabolic health and sleep apnea, focusing on how metabolic dysregulation contributes to the severity of the condition and how it interacts with sleep disturbances. We will delve into the science behind metabolic therapies, including the use of GLP-1 receptor agonists like Zepbound and how they complement sleep implant therapy to optimize results.

Additionally, we will explore the latest advancements in combining GLP-1 therapies with sleep implant treatments, offering a holistic approach to managing both the mechanical and metabolic components of sleep apnea. By integrating these therapies, patients are not only improving their sleep quality but also addressing underlying metabolic issues, ultimately leading to better long-term outcomes and quality of life.

The case studies presented in this chapter were based on real experiences as documented by Inspire Sleep and the National Library of Medicine (US). However, to protect the privacy of individuals, all names and identifying details have been changed.

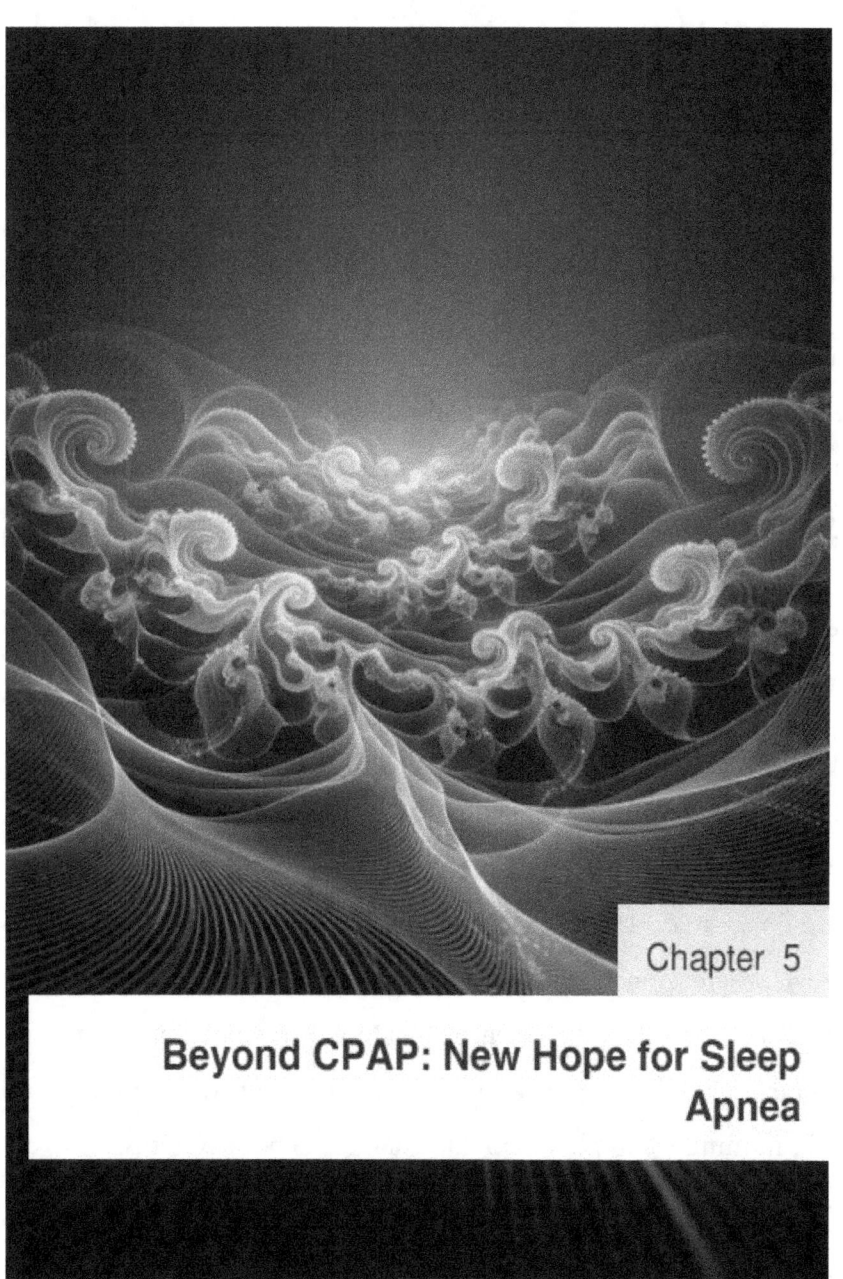

Chapter 5

Beyond CPAP: New Hope for Sleep Apnea

Chapter 5:
Metabolic Enhancement and Integrating GLP1 Therapies with Sleep Implants

Exploring Metabolic Dysregulation in Sleep Apnea

Imagine your metabolism and your breathing during sleep as two interconnected neighbors, constantly shaping each other's behavior. When one neighbor (your metabolism) starts acting out of sync, it's only a matter of time before the other neighbor (your breathing during sleep) is affected. Sleep apnea and metabolic disorders don't merely exist side by side—they have a dynamic, reciprocal relationship that amplifies each other's impact.

When we discuss metabolic dysregulation, we're delving into disturbances in how your body manages energy. This includes disruptions in insulin function, fat storage, and hormonal balance. These imbalances don't just emerge from sleep apnea—they can also fuel its progression, creating a vicious cycle where each condition exacerbates the other. In essence, metabolic dysfunction can trigger sleep apnea, while the presence of sleep apnea can worsen metabolic health, forming a complex loop that challenges both systems.

Let's break down this relationship:

How metabolic issues worsen sleep apnea:

- Fat deposition in the upper airway physically narrows breathing passages
- Reduced lung volume due to abdominal fat pressing against the diaphragm
- Inflammation from metabolic disorders causes swelling in airway tissues
- Altered respiratory control due to hormonal changes from insulin resistance

How sleep apnea disrupts metabolism:

- Intermittent hypoxia (oxygen drops) triggers insulin resistance
- Sleep fragmentation disrupts hunger hormones (increasing ghrelin and decreasing leptin)
- Stress hormone surges from breathing interruptions raise blood sugar
- Disrupted circadian rhythms affect metabolic functions throughout the body

The Obesity Connection: More than Just Weight

While many people understand that excess weight can contribute to sleep apnea, the relationship is more complex than simply having extra tissue in the throat. Obesity creates a state of chronic, low-grade inflammation throughout the body that directly impacts breathing during sleep.

When excess fat accumulates, particularly around the abdomen and neck, it doesn't just sit there passively. This tissue actively releases inflammatory compounds called cytokines that create systemic inflammation. This inflammation affects the tissues in your airway, making them more prone to collapse during sleep.

Additionally, fat cells affect your body's response to leptin, a hormone that normally helps regulate appetite and energy expenditure. In many people with obesity, the body becomes resistant to leptin's signals, creating a cascade of hormonal imbalances that further disrupt metabolism and breathing control.

Impact of Weight Loss on Sleep Apnea and Implants

When we carry excess weight, especially around the neck and abdomen, it sets the stage for a perfect storm that exacerbates sleep apnea. Extra fat around the neck narrows the upper airway, making it harder for air to flow freely. Meanwhile, abdominal fat presses against the diaphragm, limiting lung capacity and making it more difficult to take in a full breath. It's like trying to breathe through a straw that's been pinched, all while something heavy is resting on your chest—straining both your breathing and your body's ability to get the oxygen it needs. This combination can trigger or worsen sleep apnea, making each breath feel like a struggle.

Weight loss directly counteracts these mechanical challenges. For many patients, a 10-15% reduction in body weight can lead to a remarkable 50% decrease in sleep apnea severity. This improvement occurs because:

- Reduced neck circumference creates more space in the upper airway
- Decreased tongue size (yes, tongues can store fat too!)
- Lower abdominal pressure on the diaphragm improves breathing mechanics
- Reduced tissue inflammation throughout the respiratory system

Did you know?

A 2024 study published in *The Journal of Clinical Endocrinology & Metabolism* reinforced the strong link between weight loss and sleep apnea improvement. The research cited data showing that a 10% reduction in body weight led to a 26% decrease in the apnea-hypopnea index (AHI), a key measure of sleep apnea severity. Additionally, patients who underwent bariatric surgery achieved OSA remission in up to 65% of cases, highlighting the potential for substantial weight loss to improve or even resolve sleep apnea significantly.

How Weight Loss Enhances Sleep Implant Effectiveness

For patients with sleep implants like hypoglossal nerve stimulators (discussed in Chapter 3), weight loss creates a powerful synergistic effect. The implant works by stimulating the tongue to move forward during sleep, keeping the airway open. When combined with weight loss, this effect becomes more pronounced for several reasons:

- Reduced tissue volume means the implant needs to overcome less resistance

- Lower inflammatory burden creates more responsive airway tissues
- Improved metabolic health enhances overall sleep architecture
- Better oxygen utilization reduces the frequency of breathing events

Sustainable Weight Loss Strategies for Sleep Apnea Patients

Achieving meaningful weight loss isn't about quick fixes—it's about sustainable lifestyle changes that address the unique challenges sleep apnea patients face. Sleep deprivation, hormonal imbalances, and daytime fatigue can all contribute to difficulties in managing weight. Therefore, a targeted, science-backed approach is essential for long-term success. Here are evidence-based strategies that work particularly well for people with sleep apnea:

- Prioritize protein-rich foods: High-protein meals help preserve muscle mass during weight loss and increase satiety, reducing overall calorie intake. For sleep apnea patients, who often struggle with fatigue-driven food cravings and blood sugar fluctuations, protein can be especially helpful in maintaining stable energy levels throughout the day. Lean meats, fish, eggs, legumes, and dairy products are excellent protein sources.

Consider timing-based eating approaches: Many sleep apnea patients benefit from time-restricted eating (a form of intermittent fasting), which can help regulate circadian rhythms, support metabolic health, and improve sleep patterns. Eating within a structured time window—such as an 8—to 10-hour period during the day—may help reduce nighttime acid reflux, which is commonly linked to both sleep apnea and obesity.

Reduce processed carbohydrate intake: Diets high in refined carbohydrates and sugars can lead to insulin resistance, increased fat storage, and worsened inflammation—all of which are risk factors for obesity and sleep apnea. Replacing processed foods with whole grains, vegetables, and fiber-rich alternatives can help stabilize blood sugar and reduce excess weight gain.

- Increase anti-inflammatory foods: Chronic inflammation contributes to weight gain and airway obstruction. Incorporating foods rich in omega-3 fatty acids (such as fatty fish, flaxseeds, and walnuts), antioxidants (berries, leafy greens), and polyphenols (green tea, dark chocolate) can help reduce systemic inflammation and support better sleep quality.

Stay physically active—even with low energy: Daytime fatigue can make exercise difficult for sleep apnea patients, but movement is essential for weight management and sleep quality. Low-impact activities such as walking, swimming, cycling, and yoga can be effective without exacerbating exhaustion. Strength training can also help maintain muscle mass, which supports a higher resting metabolic rate.

- Prioritize sleep hygiene to support weight loss: Poor sleep disrupts hormones that regulate appetite—specifically, increasing ghrelin (the hunger hormone) and decreasing leptin (the satiety hormone). Establishing a consistent bedtime routine, limiting screen exposure before bed, and optimizing sleep environment conditions (cool, dark, and quiet) can improve sleep quality and help regulate appetite.

Manage stress and emotional eating: Sleep apnea and obesity are both linked to high stress levels, which can trigger emotional eating and increased cortisol production, leading to weight gain. Mindfulness practices, relaxation techniques, and structured meal planning can help patients make healthier food choices.

Definition and Mechanism of GLP-1 Receptor Agonists

To understand GLP-1 receptor agonists, let's first look at what happens naturally in your body. When you eat, your intestines release a hormone called glucagon-like peptide-1 (GLP-1). Think of GLP-1 as your body's built-in appetite controller and metabolism manager. It travels through your bloodstream, delivering several important messages:

- To your brain: "You've eaten enough—feel satisfied."
- To your stomach: "Slow down digestion so nutrients are absorbed gradually."
- To your pancreas: "Release insulin to handle the incoming nutrients."

GLP-1 receptor agonists are medications that mimic this natural hormone but with enhanced strength and duration. They're like a longer-lasting, more powerful version of your body's own GLP-1, binding to the same receptors and triggering the same beneficial effects.

Did you know?

A 2022 study published in the New England Journal of Medicine found that patients taking semaglutide, a GLP-1 receptor agonist, experienced an average weight loss of 15% over 68 weeks—substantially higher than the 2.4% lost in the placebo group. Notably, this weight loss was predominantly from fat tissue, rather than muscle mass, highlighting the drug's potential to target fat while preserving lean body mass. This makes semaglutide an especially promising option for those looking to manage weight more effectively, without the risk of muscle loss typically associated with other weight loss methods.

How GLP-1 Agonists Work: A Multi-System Approach

GLP-1 receptor agonists work through several mechanisms simultaneously, creating a comprehensive approach to metabolic regulation:

Brain Effects: Appetite Control

These medications target the hypothalamus—your brain's hunger control center—and areas involved in food reward and craving. By activating GLP-1 receptors in these regions, they:

- Reduce hunger signals
- Increase feelings of fullness
- Decrease the pleasure response to high-calorie foods
- Help you feel satisfied with smaller portions

Digestive System: Slowing Things Down

GLP-1 agonists significantly slow gastric emptying—the rate at which food leaves your stomach and enters your small intestine. This creates several beneficial effects:

- Food stays in your stomach longer, maintaining fullness
- Nutrients are absorbed more gradually, preventing blood sugar spikes
- You naturally eat less because you feel satisfied longer

Introduction to Zepbound as an Adjunct Therapy

Zepbound (tirzepatide) represents a significant breakthrough in GLP-1 therapy. While earlier medications in this class primarily targeted GLP-1 receptors, Zepbound works as a dual GIP and GLP-1 receptor agonist, which means it activates two different hormone pathways instead of just one.

Think of it like having two different keys that unlock complementary doors in your metabolism. The GLP-1 component works as we discussed in the previous section—controlling appetite, slowing digestion, and improving insulin sensitivity. The added GIP (glucose-dependent insulinotropic polypeptide) activation enhances these effects while providing additional benefits:

- More powerful weight loss than single-target GLP-1 medications
- Greater improvements in insulin sensitivity and glucose control

- Enhanced fat metabolism throughout the body
- Reduced inflammatory markers associated with sleep apnea

Did you know?

In the groundbreaking SURMOUNT-OSA clinical trials completed in 2023, participants taking Zepbound experienced a remarkable 25-29 fewer breathing disruptions per hour compared to only 5-6 fewer disruptions in the placebo group. This dramatic improvement occurred whether patients were using PAP therapy or not.

Zepbound and Sleep Implants: A Powerful Combination

While Zepbound was initially approved for weight management and later for sleep apnea, sleep specialists quickly recognized its potential as a complementary therapy for patients with sleep implants. The combination addresses sleep apnea through different but synergistic mechanisms:

- Sleep implants directly stimulate airway muscles to maintain patency during sleep
- Zepbound addresses the underlying metabolic factors that contribute to airway collapse

Beyond Weight Loss: Metabolic Benefits for Sleep Apnea

While the weight loss Zepbound produces (typically 15-20% of body weight) certainly helps sleep apnea, its benefits extend beyond simply shedding pounds. Research suggests that Zepbound improves sleep apnea through several additional mechanisms:

- Reduced systemic inflammation that contributes to airway tissue swelling
- Improved fat distribution with greater loss of visceral fat that affects breathing mechanics
- Enhanced respiratory muscle function through improved metabolic health
- Better sleep architecture through stabilized blood sugar during the night

For patients with sleep implants, these metabolic improvements provide a holistic approach to managing sleep apnea, enhancing both immediate and long-term outcomes.

Effectiveness and Mechanics of Zepbound

What makes Zepbound (tirzepatide) particularly effective for sleep apnea patients is its unique dual-action approach. Unlike earlier medications that target only one pathway, Zepbound activates two complementary hormone receptors:

- GLP-1 receptors (glucagon-like peptide-1): Control appetite, slow digestion, and improve insulin sensitivity
- GIP receptors (glucose-dependent insulinotropic polypeptide): Enhance fat metabolism and further improve metabolic function

This dual activation creates a more powerful effect than either pathway alone. Think of it like rowing a boat with two oars instead of one—you move faster and with better control.

How Zepbound Transforms Breathing during Sleep

Zepbound improves sleep breathing through several interconnected mechanisms:

Significant Weight Loss

The most visible effect of Zepbound is substantial weight reduction. In clinical trials, patients lost an average of 18-20% of their body weight (about 45-50 pounds for many participants). This weight loss directly impacts sleep apnea by:

- Reducing fat deposits around the neck and throat that compress the airway
- Decreasing abdominal fat that limits diaphragm movement during breathing
- Lightening the overall load on the respiratory system

Reduced Airway Inflammation

Beyond weight loss, Zepbound reduces systemic inflammation throughout the body. This is crucial for sleep apnea patients, as inflammation in airway tissues contributes significantly to nighttime breathing problems. By lowering inflammatory markers like C-reactive protein, Zepbound helps create less swollen, more flexible airway tissues that are less likely to collapse during sleep.

Improved Sleep Architecture

Zepbound stabilizes blood sugar levels throughout the night, which helps maintain more consistent sleep patterns. Many sleep apnea patients experience blood sugar fluctuations that fragment sleep, even when their breathing is supported. By smoothing these metabolic fluctuations, Zepbound helps patients spend more time in restorative deep sleep and REM sleep stages.

Enhanced Respiratory Control

The GLP-1 component of Zepbound appears to improve the brain's respiratory control centers. Research suggests it may help stabilize breathing patterns beyond what can be explained by weight loss alone, potentially through direct effects on brainstem regions that regulate breathing during sleep.

Review of Clinical Studies on GLP-1 in Sleep Apnea

The landscape of sleep apnea treatment changed dramatically with the SURMOUNT-OSA clinical trials, which examined tirzepatide (Zepbound) specifically for sleep apnea. These landmark studies divided participants into two groups—those using PAP therapy and those not using it—to determine if GLP-1 therapy could make a meaningful difference.

The results were nothing short of remarkable:

- Participants taking Zepbound experienced 25-29 fewer breathing disruptions per hour (compared to just 5-6 fewer in the placebo group)
- 42-50% of participants achieved either complete remission of their sleep apnea or improved to only mild, non-symptomatic OSA

- Benefits were observed regardless of whether patients were using PAP therapy

These findings led to the historic FDA approval of tirzepatide (Zepbound) in December 2024 as the first medication specifically indicated for treating moderate-to-severe obstructive sleep apnea in adults with obesity—a watershed moment in sleep medicine.

Beyond Zepbound: The Broader GLP-1 Evidence Base

While Zepbound has garnered the most attention, other GLP-1 receptor agonists have also shown promising results for sleep apnea:

- Semaglutide (Wegovy/Ozempic): Multiple studies show significant reductions in AHI, with one trial documenting an average 20-point decrease in participants with moderate-to-severe OSA
- Liraglutide (Saxenda): A case report documented an AHI reduction from 27 to 7.1 events per hour—moving a patient from moderate to mild sleep apnea
- Dulaglutide (Trulicity): Emerging data suggests improvements in sleep quality and reduced daytime sleepiness in patients with type 2 diabetes and OSA

Mechanisms beyond Weight Loss

Perhaps the most fascinating aspect of the research is that GLP-1 therapies appear to improve sleep apnea through multiple mechanisms—not just weight loss. Studies examining the timing of improvements have found that some patients experience better sleep quality before significant weight reduction occurs.

Research published by Dragonieri and colleagues in 2024 identified several weight-independent mechanisms:

- Anti-inflammatory effects: GLP-1 therapies reduce systemic inflammation, decreasing swelling in airway tissues
- Improved respiratory control: GLP-1 receptors in the central nervous system help stabilize breathing patterns during sleep
- Enhanced upper airway muscle function: Metabolic benefits that contribute to improved muscle tone and function

These findings underscore the potential of GLP-1 therapies to revolutionize sleep apnea treatment, offering hope for patients who struggle with traditional interventions.

GLP-1 and Implant Therapy

Emerging clinical data suggests that combining GLP-1 therapies with sleep implants creates a powerful synergy that exceeds what either treatment can achieve alone. While research specifically examining this combination is still developing, early clinical observations and case series show remarkable patterns of improvement.

The combined approach appears to work through complementary mechanisms:

- Sleep implants: Provide immediate mechanical support to keep airways open during sleep.

- GLP-1 therapies: Address the underlying metabolic factors that contribute to airway collapse.

Did you know?

A 2023 analysis from the Cleveland Clinic Journal of Medicine assessed the effectiveness of hypoglossal nerve stimulation (HNS) in patients with obstructive sleep apnea (OSA). The study found that HNS significantly improved apnea-hypopnea index (AHI) scores, with success rates as high as 81.5% in patients with independent epiglottic collapse.

Measurable Improvements in Sleep Parameters

When we look at specific sleep measurements, the combination of GLP-1 therapies and sleep implants shows impressive improvements across multiple parameters:

- Apnea-Hypopnea Index (AHI): Combined therapy typically reduces breathing events by 65-80% from baseline, compared to 50-60% with implants alone.
- Oxygen Saturation: Patients show higher average overnight oxygen levels and fewer desaturation events.
- Sleep Architecture: More time spent in restorative deep sleep and REM sleep phases.
- Sleep Efficiency: Less fragmented sleep with fewer arousals and awakenings.

These improvements translate into tangible benefits that patients notice in their daily lives—often within weeks of starting combination therapy.

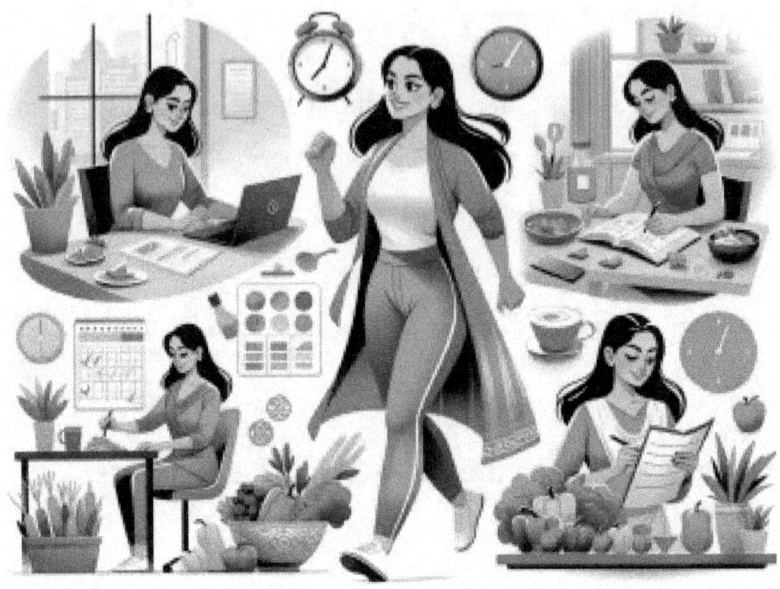

Illustration: A person engaging in daily activities with increased energy and alertness.

Quality of Life Transformations

While clinical measurements are important, the real impact of combined therapy is best understood through patient-reported outcomes. In quality of life assessments, patients consistently receiving both treatments report dramatic improvements in:

- Daytime alertness: "I no longer need afternoon naps just to get through the day."
- Cognitive function: "My brain fog has lifted—I can focus at work again."

- Mood stability: "I'm less irritable and more patient with my family."
- Physical energy: "I have the energy to exercise now, which helps me lose even more weight."
- Relationship satisfaction: "My partner says I'm a different person."

These transformations highlight the profound impact that combined GLP-1 and implant therapy can have on patients' lives.

Developing Integrative Treatment Protocols

Creating an effective integrated protocol isn't simply prescribing two treatments simultaneously—it requires thoughtful coordination and monitoring. Based on emerging clinical experience and research, several key components have proven essential:

- Comprehensive baseline assessment of both sleep parameters and metabolic health
- Strategic timing of when to introduce each therapy component
- Regular monitoring with appropriate adjustments to optimize outcomes
- Supportive lifestyle modifications that enhance both treatments

Step-by-Step Protocol Development

While protocols must be tailored to individual patient needs, a general framework has emerged that provides structure for healthcare providers:

Comprehensive Initial Assessment

Before beginning combined therapy, patients should undergo:

- Complete sleep study (polysomnography or home sleep apnea testing)
- Metabolic evaluation, including body composition analysis
- Airway assessment to understand structural factors
- Evaluation of current symptoms and quality of life measures

Establish Treatment Sequence

Determining whether to start with the implant or GLP-1 therapy depends on several factors:

- Implant first approach: Often preferred for patients with severe sleep apnea requiring immediate intervention
- GLP-1 first approach: May be appropriate for patients with mild-to-moderate apnea and significant obesity
- Simultaneous initiation: Sometimes used when both interventions are urgently needed

Implement Continuous Monitoring

Unlike traditional approaches that might check progress every 6-12 months, integrated protocols typically include:

- Monthly assessments during the first three months
- Objective sleep monitoring using home testing devices
- Regular evaluation of implant settings as weight changes occur
- Tracking of metabolic markers alongside sleep parameters

Coordinate Supportive Care

Effective protocols include support systems that enhance both treatments:

- Nutritional guidance specific to GLP-1 therapy
- Exercise programs tailored to improve metabolic health and sleep quality
- Behavioral therapy to support lifestyle changes

Patient Selection and Treatment Personalization

Not every sleep apnea patient will benefit equally from combined GLP-1 and implant therapy. Identifying the right candidates involves a thoughtful assessment of multiple factors. The most promising candidates typically share several key characteristics:

- Persistent sleep apnea symptoms despite having a functional sleep implant
- BMI over 30 (or over 27 with weight-related health conditions)
- Central adiposity with significant neck circumference
- Signs of metabolic dysfunction such as insulin resistance or prediabetes
- History of weight-related breathing difficulties
- Motivation to make complementary lifestyle changes

Did you know?

A 2023 analysis from the Cleveland Clinic Journal of Medicine and other research suggests that integrating weight loss strategies with sleep apnea treatments can significantly improve outcomes, particularly for patients with a BMI over 32 and moderate-to-severe OSA (AHI >15). Studies indicate that GLP-1 receptor agonists, such as semaglutide, not only promote weight loss but also reduce the apnea-hypopnea index (AHI) beyond what is typically seen with standard therapies.

Personalization Factors That Enhance Success

Beyond simply identifying suitable candidates, truly effective treatment requires personalization based on individual patient characteristics. Several key factors should guide treatment customization:

Sleep Apnea Phenotype

Not all sleep apnea is created equal. Patients exhibit different "phenotypes" or patterns of breathing disruption:

- Anatomical obstruction: Primarily caused by physical narrowing of the airway
- Muscle tone issues: Related to reduced neuromuscular control during sleep
- Arousal threshold problems: Overly sensitive awakening response to minor breathing changes
- Mixed patterns: Combinations of multiple underlying mechanisms

Understanding a patient's specific phenotype helps determine how much they might benefit from metabolic intervention alongside their implant therapy.

Metabolic Health Assessment

A comprehensive metabolic evaluation provides crucial insights for treatment personalization:

- Body composition analysis: Understanding fat distribution patterns
- Insulin sensitivity testing: Identifying insulin resistance
- Inflammatory markers: Assessing systemic inflammation
- Lipid profiles: Evaluating cardiovascular risk factors

Addressing Potential Challenges and Benefits

While integrating GLP-1 therapies with sleep implants offers tremendous potential, several challenges must be addressed to ensure treatment success:

Side Effect Management

GLP-1 therapies commonly cause gastrointestinal side effects, particularly during the initial weeks of treatment. These can include:

- Nausea and vomiting, especially after eating larger meals
- Delayed gastric emptying causing fullness and occasional discomfort
- Diarrhea or constipation as the digestive system adapts

Cost and Access Barriers

Perhaps the most significant challenge for many patients is the financial burden of combined therapy:

- GLP-1 medications can cost $900-$1,300 per month without insurance coverage
- Many insurance plans classify these medications as "weight loss drugs" rather than sleep apnea treatments
- Prior authorization requirements create administrative hurdles

Healthcare providers are addressing these challenges through several approaches:

- Advocating with insurance companies using sleep study data to demonstrate medical necessity
- Connecting patients with manufacturer assistance programs
- Documenting improvements in multiple health parameters to support continued coverage

Coordination of Care Challenges

Effective combined therapy requires seamless coordination between multiple specialists:

- Sleep medicine physicians managing implant settings
- Endocrinologists or primary care providers overseeing GLP-1 therapy
- Dietitians providing nutritional support
- Mental health professionals addressing psychological aspects of treatment

Strategies to Enhance Treatment Success

Despite these challenges, several evidence-based strategies have emerged to improve outcomes in combined therapy. By optimizing treatment adherence, minimizing side effects, and fostering interdisciplinary collaboration, patients can achieve better long-term results.

Gradual Dose Adjustments and Dietary Modifications

A structured approach to GLP-1 therapy initiation is recommended to minimize gastrointestinal discomfort:

- Slow titration: Gradually increasing the medication dose over several weeks allows the body to adjust, reducing the likelihood of severe nausea or vomiting.
- Smaller, more frequent meals: Patients are encouraged to eat nutrient-dense, smaller meals to accommodate slower gastric emptying without causing excessive fullness.

Avoiding trigger foods: Greasy, highly processed, or excessively sugary foods can worsen side effects and should be limited.

- Hydration and fiber intake: Staying well-hydrated and consuming adequate fiber can help prevent constipation, a common issue with GLP-1 therapy.

Maximizing Insurance Coverage and Financial Assistance

Given the high cost of GLP-1 medications, patients and healthcare providers can explore several avenues to improve affordability:

- Appealing insurance denials: Submitting sleep study data and physician reports can strengthen the case for coverage.

- Using patient assistance programs: Some pharmaceutical companies offer discount programs or financial aid for eligible patients.
- Exploring compounded medications: In some cases, compounding pharmacies provide lower-cost versions of GLP-1 medications, though quality and availability vary.

Personalized Therapy Adjustments

Because each patient responds differently to treatment, ongoing monitoring, and tailored adjustments are critical for success:

Optimizing implant settings: Sleep medicine specialists can fine-tune the stimulation parameters to maximize airway support while minimizing discomfort.

- Tracking metabolic changes: Regular lab tests to monitor glucose levels, lipid profiles, and body composition can help assess treatment efficacy.
- Behavioral support: Incorporating psychological counseling or cognitive behavioral therapy (CBT) for emotional eating and motivation can enhance adherence to lifestyle changes.

Long-Term Monitoring and Lifestyle Integration

Patients benefit most when treatment is integrated into a broader lifestyle approach that includes:

- Regular sleep assessments: Follow-up sleep studies can ensure that implant therapy remains effective as weight loss progresses.

Exercise and strength training: Maintaining muscle mass is essential for metabolic health and sustained weight management.

- Ongoing dietary guidance: As weight loss occurs, nutritional needs change, requiring periodic adjustments from a registered dietitian.

Conclusion and Transition

In Chapter 5, we explored the synergistic potential of combining GLP-1 therapies with sleep implants for managing sleep apnea. By addressing both the mechanical airway issues through sleep implants and the underlying metabolic disruptions through GLP-1 medications, this integrative approach has shown promising results in improving sleep quality, reducing apnea events, and enhancing overall health. As demonstrated through patient experiences, the combination of weight loss, metabolic regulation, and sleep therapy can result in profound transformations in both sleep apnea severity and daytime energy levels. This holistic treatment method not only improves sleep outcomes but also addresses the root causes of the condition, making it a comprehensive solution for many patients.

In Chapter 6, we will explore the latest advancements in sleep apnea management, particularly focusing on the integration of biomarker-driven diagnostics and advanced pharmacological approaches. As we transition from the mechanical treatments discussed in previous chapters to a more personalized and holistic approach, we'll look at how biomarkers like microRNAs are revolutionizing diagnosis and treatment selection, allowing for more accurate and tailored interventions.

Additionally, we will delve into the growing role of pharmacological therapies, particularly GLP-1 receptor agonists, in complementing traditional treatments like sleep implants. These medications, which address underlying metabolic factors such as obesity, are proving to be powerful allies in the fight against sleep apnea.

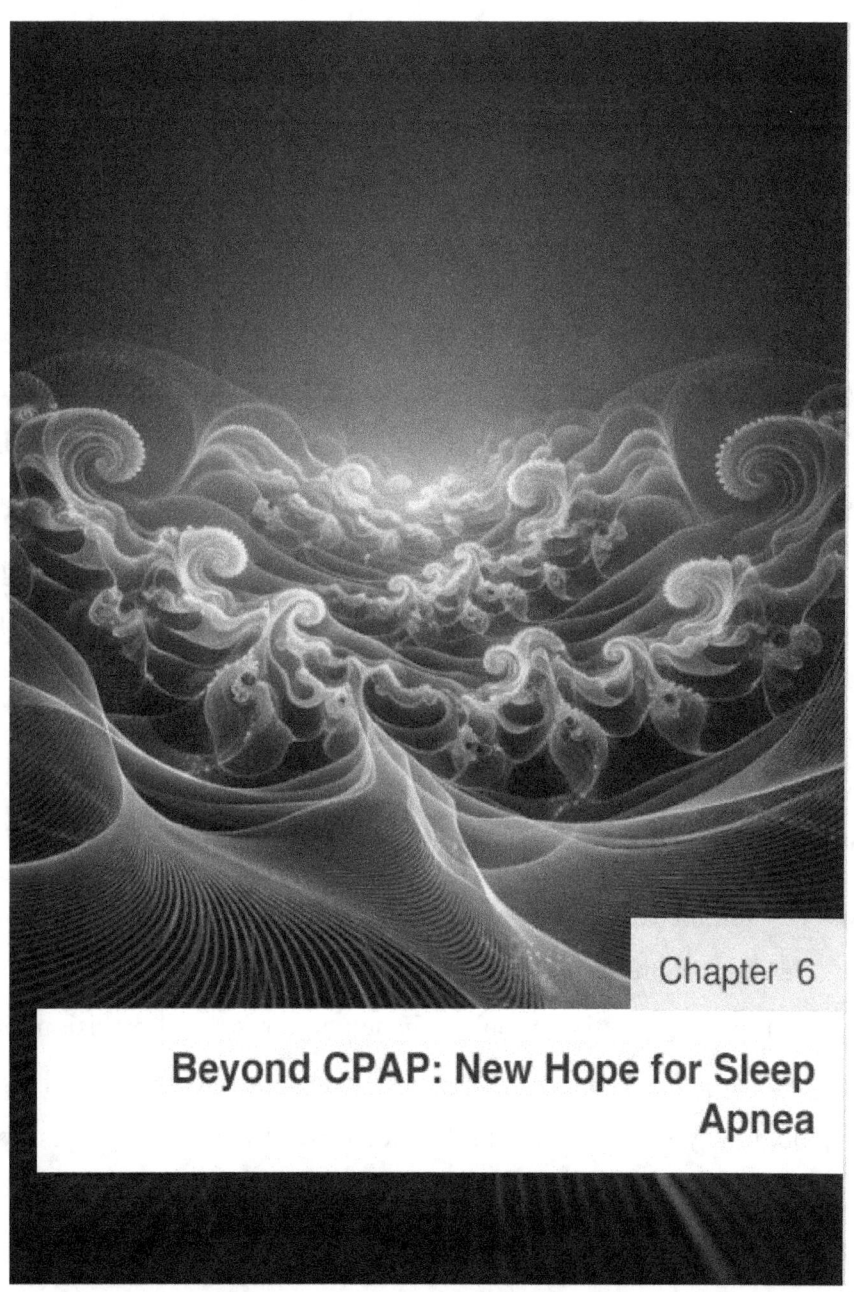

Chapter 6

Beyond CPAP: New Hope for Sleep Apnea

Chapter 6:
Innovations and Future Directions

Reimagining Sleep Apnea Treatment

Imagine a future where your sleep apnea treatment doesn't just react to your breathing but actually learns from it—adapting in real-time, predicting problems before they happen, and adjusting to your unique sleep patterns without you lifting a finger. That future isn't far off. In fact, it's already unfolding.

In this chapter, we turn our gaze forward to explore the cutting-edge innovations reshaping the world of sleep apnea treatment. From AI-driven neurostimulation systems and miniaturized implants to genetic insights and personalized medicine, the field is evolving rapidly—and patients are starting to benefit in ways we couldn't have imagined just a decade ago.

We'll examine how next-generation devices are getting smaller, smarter, and more in sync with your body. You will discover how artificial intelligence is not only enhancing comfort and precision but also reducing the need for constant in-person adjustments. We will also explore how your DNA might influence which therapies work best for you and how global market shifts are accelerating access to these revolutionary solutions.

As the world of sleep medicine evolves, one thing is clear: the future is personalized, predictive, and profoundly patient-centered. Let's dive into the innovations leading the way.

Neurostimulation Devices

Neurostimulation devices represent one of the most significant breakthroughs in sleep apnea treatment since CPAP therapy. These implantable technologies offer a completely different approach to keeping airways open during sleep—working with your body's natural systems rather than forcing air through your airway.

How Neurostimulation Works

The most widely used neurostimulation device for sleep apnea is the hypoglossal nerve stimulator (HNS). This clever system works by gently stimulating the nerve that controls your tongue (the hypoglossal nerve), causing it to move slightly forward during sleep. This subtle movement prevents your tongue from falling back and blocking your airway—the primary cause of obstructive sleep apnea in many people.

Think of it as having a helpful friend who gently nudges your tongue forward every time you breathe in while sleeping. The system consists of three main parts:

- A small pulse generator implanted under the skin in your upper chest (similar in size to a pacemaker)
- A breathing sensor lead placed between your ribs to detect your breathing pattern
- A stimulation lead connected to your hypoglossal nerve under your chin

What makes this technology truly remarkable is its intelligent design. The system monitors your breathing patterns and delivers stimulation only when needed. When you inhale during sleep, the device sends a gentle pulse to your hypoglossal nerve, moving your tongue forward and opening your airway. When you exhale, the stimulation pauses. This synchronized approach means the therapy works only when you're sleeping and only when you need it.

Did you know?

A 2022 study published in the *Journal of Clinical Sleep Medicine* found that patients using hypoglossal nerve stimulation (HNS) experienced significant reductions in sleep apnea severity. Research on HNS has demonstrated substantial improvements in the apnea-hypopnea index (AHI), with studies showing reductions of around 50–68% in appropriately selected patients. These findings highlight the effectiveness of HNS as a treatment option for obstructive sleep apnea (OSA), particularly for individuals who struggle with CPAP adherence.

The Inspire System: Leading the Revolution

The most established neurostimulation device is the Inspire Upper Airway Stimulation system, which received FDA approval in 2014 and has since helped thousands of patients worldwide. The latest generation of this device is smaller, more efficient, and lasts longer than early models.

What makes the Inspire system particularly user-friendly is its remote control. Before going to sleep, you simply press a button on a small remote to activate the device. Another press turns it off when you wake up. Some newer models even allow you to adjust the stimulation strength to find your most comfortable setting.

The implantation procedure typically takes about two hours under general anesthesia. Most patients go home the same day and return to normal activities within a week or two. The device isn't activated immediately—most doctors wait about a month for healing before turning it on and adjusting the settings to their specific needs.

AI-Driven Therapy Customization

Artificial intelligence is transforming sleep implant therapy by offering a level of personalization never seen before. Unlike traditional devices, which rely on fixed settings, AI-powered implants continuously monitor your sleep data and make real-time adjustments to ensure the therapy is tailored to your unique needs. This dynamic approach allows the device to respond immediately to changes in your sleep patterns, delivering precise treatment exactly when it's needed, enhancing both effectiveness and comfort. It's a major leap forward in providing more adaptive and responsive care for sleep disorders.

Real-Time Adaptation

The most significant advantage of AI-driven implants is their ability to adapt therapy in real-time. Traditional implants deliver consistent stimulation based on settings determined during occasional doctor visits. AI-enhanced devices, however, monitor hundreds of variables throughout the night and adjust accordingly.

- Enter different sleep stages (REM vs. deep sleep)
- Change sleeping positions
- Experience variations in breathing patterns
- Have episodes of increased airway resistance

Based on this information, the device automatically adjusts stimulation intensity, timing, and pattern. If you roll onto your back—a position that typically worsens sleep apnea—the system might increase stimulation strength. During REM sleep, when apnea events often become more frequent, the device can deliver more precisely timed pulses.

Learning From Your Sleep Patterns

What makes these systems truly remarkable is their ability to learn from your unique sleep patterns over time. The implant uses sophisticated machine learning algorithms to analyze weeks of data to identify patterns specific to you:

For instance, if the AI notices that you consistently experience more severe apnea events around 3 AM, it might preemptively increase stimulation shortly before that time. Or if it recognizes that your breathing becomes more regular after certain stimulation patterns, it will favor those patterns in similar situations.

Personalized Therapy without Doctor Visits

Traditional implants require multiple in-office visits for adjustments as your condition changes or if you're not getting optimal results. AI-driven systems can make many of these adjustments automatically, reducing the need for frequent appointments.

These smart-systems also provide valuable insights to your healthcare team. When you visit your doctor, they can review detailed reports showing how your therapy has been automatically optimized. This data helps inform any manual adjustments that might still be beneficial.

Miniaturization and Design Innovations

The evolution of sleep apnea implants mirrors what we've seen with many technologies—from room-sized computers to smartphones, medical devices are following a similar trajectory toward smaller, smarter, and more user-friendly designs. This miniaturization revolution is transforming sleep apnea treatment by making implants less invasive, more comfortable, and increasingly effective.

The Shrinking Footprint

Early sleep implants were groundbreaking in concept but bulky in execution. The first FDA-approved hypoglossal nerve stimulator resembled a pacemaker in size and required substantial surgical space for implantation. Today's devices tell a different story:

- Reduced implant size: Newer models are up to 60% smaller than first-generation devices
- Thinner profiles: Modern implants protrude less beneath the skin, making them nearly invisible after healing
- Smaller incisions: Less invasive surgical techniques reduce scarring and recovery time
- Streamlined components: Integration of previously separate parts into single units

The Inspire V system exemplifies this trend, incorporating sensing functions directly into the neurostimulator—reducing the number of components surgeons need to implant. This integration not only makes the device smaller but also shortens the procedure time from 60-90 minutes to 45-60 minutes.

Material Innovations Driving Change

The dramatic reduction in implant size wouldn't be possible without parallel advances in materials science. Today's devices leverage several cutting-edge materials:

- Biocompatible polymers: Lightweight casings that cause minimal tissue reaction
- Titanium alloys: Stronger yet lighter metal components that resist corrosion
- Flexible circuitry: Bendable electronic components that conform to body contours

- Advanced battery chemistry: Smaller power sources that maintain or extend device longevity

Power Efficiency: Doing More with Less

Perhaps the most impressive aspect of miniaturization is that these smaller devices actually last longer than their larger predecessors. This seemingly magical feat comes from dramatic improvements in power management:

- Low-power microprocessors: Using less energy while performing more complex functions
- Adaptive stimulation: Delivering therapy only when needed rather than continuously, conserving energy
- Smart battery management: Extending battery life through efficient power use

These advancements ensure that patients benefit from longer-lasting, more reliable devices that enhance their quality of life without frequent maintenance or replacement.

Introduction to Personalized Medicine

Traditional sleep apnea treatment has followed a relatively standardized pathway: diagnosis via a sleep study, followed by CPAP therapy as the first-line treatment, with alternatives like oral appliances or surgery for those who can't tolerate CPAP. While this approach helps many patients, it leaves others struggling with suboptimal outcomes or abandoning treatment altogether.

Personalized medicine takes a fundamentally different approach by recognizing that sleep apnea is not a single disorder but a spectrum of conditions with varying causes, presentations, and optimal treatment paths. Rather than starting every patient on the same treatment journey, personalized medicine asks: "What specific factors are driving this individual's sleep apnea, and which targeted interventions will work best for their unique situation?"

Several converging factors are driving this shift toward personalization:

- Advances in diagnostic technology that can pinpoint specific causes of airway obstruction
- Growing understanding of sleep apnea subtypes and their varying responses to different treatments
- Emerging research on genetic factors that influence both sleep apnea development and treatment response
- The integration of AI and machine learning to analyze complex patient data and identify optimal treatment pathways

Role of AI in Personalized Treatment

Artificial intelligence is revolutionizing sleep apnea treatment by transforming standard implants into sophisticated systems that learn, adapt, and optimize therapy based on your unique needs. This personalization goes far beyond the one-size-fits-all approach of traditional treatments.

Just as your fingerprint is unique, your sleep patterns have distinctive characteristics that AI can identify and analyze. Modern AI-powered implants collect data on hundreds of variables during your sleep:

- Breathing patterns: The rhythm, depth, and variability of your breathing
- Sleep architecture: Your transitions between different sleep stages
- Body position: How your sleep apnea changes when you sleep on your back versus your side
- Response patterns: How your airway responds to different levels of stimulation

Over time, the AI builds what sleep scientists call your "sleep fingerprint"—a comprehensive profile of your unique sleep characteristics. This profile allows the system to predict when apnea events are likely to occur and determine the most effective response for your specific physiology.

Dynamic Treatment Adjustment

Traditional implants use static settings determined during occasional doctor visits. AI-enhanced systems, however, continuously refine therapy in real-time based on how your body responds.

For example, if the AI detects that your breathing becomes more irregular during REM sleep, it might increase stimulation during those periods. Or if it notices that a certain stimulation pattern works particularly well for you in a specific sleep position, it will favor that pattern whenever you adopt that position.

Perhaps the most impressive capability of AI-enhanced implants is their ability to *predict* problems before they occur. Rather than simply reacting to apnea events after they start, these systems can anticipate them based on subtle changes in your breathing patterns.

Genetic Data and Treatment Optimization

Recent research has shown that genetic factors account for 35-40% of the variance in obstructive sleep apnea (OSA), as highlighted in a study by Li et al. (2020). This genetic component helps explain why sleep apnea often runs in families and why certain treatments work better for some patients than others. For instance, genetic factors influencing airway structure, muscle tone, and fat distribution play a significant role in how OSA manifests and responds to treatment (Aasmundstad et al., 2021). These findings support the idea that a more personalized, genetically-informed approach to treatment could lead to better outcomes for patients with OSA.

Scientists have identified several gene variants associated with sleep apnea, including:

- ANGPT2: Affects blood vessel formation and stability in airway tissues
- TNFα: Influences inflammation levels in upper airway tissues
- PTGER3 and LPAR1: Impact neural control of upper airway muscles
- GPR83, ARRB1, and DRD1: Affect sleep regulation and breathing control

Matching Genetics to Treatment Options

Genetic profiling is particularly valuable when deciding between different treatment approaches for sleep apnea. For example:

- Implant selection: Certain genetic markers can predict whether you'll respond better to hypoglossal nerve stimulation or other implant types
- Medication responsiveness: Genetic variations affect how you metabolize and respond to medications that might be used alongside implant therapy
- Anatomical predispositions: Genes that influence craniofacial development can help determine which implant placement will be most effective

Predicting Treatment Response

Perhaps the most valuable application of genetic data is predicting how well you'll respond to specific treatments. This capability helps avoid the frustrating cycle of trying and abandoning ineffective therapies.

For instance, researchers have identified genetic markers that predict:

- How effectively your airway muscles will respond to specific therapies
- Your body's reaction to different treatment modalities

This predictive power allows for more targeted and effective treatment plans, reducing the time and effort spent on ineffective options.

Overview of Market Growth and Opportunities

The sleep apnea implant market is experiencing remarkable growth, creating new possibilities for patients who cannot tolerate or don't respond well to CPAP therapy. Understanding these market dynamics helps explain why certain treatments become available in different regions and how quickly innovations reach patients worldwide.

Current Market Landscape

The global sleep apnea implant market reached approximately $450 million in 2024, representing a relatively small but rapidly growing segment of the broader sleep apnea treatment industry. While CPAP devices still dominate the overall sleep apnea market, implantable technologies are gaining significant momentum.

Several factors drive this growth:

- Rising diagnosis rates of sleep apnea worldwide
- Growing awareness of the limitations of traditional CPAP therapy
- Expanding insurance coverage for implantable devices
- Technological innovations making implants smaller, more effective, and less invasive

The market currently features several key players, with Inspire Medical Systems holding the largest market share for hypoglossal nerve stimulation devices. Other significant competitors include LivaNova, Nyxoah, and ImThera Medical (acquired by LivaNova), each offering unique approaches to implantable sleep apnea therapy.

Did you know?

According to a 2024 market analysis by Future Market Insights, the sleep apnea implant segment is experiencing steady growth, driven by increasing patient demand for alternatives to CPAP therapy and expanding clinical evidence supporting implant efficacy. While CPAP devices continue to dominate the market with a higher projected growth rate, the adoption of implantable treatments is rising as patients seek more comfortable and long-term solutions for sleep apnea management.

Growth Projections and Opportunities

The future looks promising for sleep implant technologies. Market analysts project the global sleep apnea implant market to reach between $677 million and $1.3 billion by 2035, depending on various factors, including regulatory approvals, reimbursement policies, and technological advancements.

This projected growth represents a compound annual growth rate (CAGR) of 3.8% to 15.4%, significantly outpacing many other medical device segments. The wide range of projections reflects both the tremendous potential and the uncertainties in this evolving market.

Several key trends are creating exciting opportunities in this space:

Regional Market Expansion

While North America currently dominates the sleep apnea implant market (accounting for approximately 60% of global revenue), other regions are showing remarkable growth potential:

- Europe: Rapid adoption is occurring in Germany, France, and the UK, where national health systems are increasingly covering implantable therapies. Regulatory streamlining and growing physician awareness are accelerating market penetration.

Asia-Pacific: Countries such as China, Japan, and Australia represent the fastest-growing regional market, with projected growth rates exceeding 15% annually. Rising healthcare expenditures, expanding middle-class populations, and increasing diagnosis rates are key drivers.

- Latin America: Brazil and Mexico are leading the region in adoption, as improving healthcare infrastructure and awareness campaigns drive demand for advanced sleep apnea treatments.

Technological Innovations and Next-Generation Implants

Several advancements are shaping the future of sleep apnea implants, making them more effective, accessible, and patient-friendly:

- Miniaturization and Smart Implants: Next-generation implants are becoming smaller, more energy-efficient, and capable of

delivering personalized stimulation based on real-time breathing patterns.
- AI-Driven Optimization: The integration of artificial intelligence is improving therapy customization, allowing for adaptive stimulation settings based on nightly variations in sleep behavior.
- Wireless and Battery-Free Devices: Researchers are exploring wireless-powered and bioresorbable implants, which could potentially eliminate the need for battery replacements and reduce long-term maintenance.

Expanding Patient Eligibility and Awareness

Traditionally, sleep implants were reserved for patients with moderate to severe obstructive sleep apnea who could not tolerate CPAP therapy. However, shifting guidelines and evolving device capabilities are broadening the eligible patient population:

- Mild OSA Patients: Some newer-generation implants are being tested for effectiveness in patients with mild obstructive sleep apnea.
- Combination Therapy Approaches: Sleep implants are increasingly being integrated with weight loss interventions, positional therapy, and pharmacological treatments such as GLP-1 medications.
- Improved Public and Physician Awareness: Educational initiatives and direct-to-patient marketing efforts are helping

more individuals recognize sleep implants as a viable alternative to CPAP.

As these trends continue to unfold, the sleep implant market is poised for transformative growth. With expanding geographic reach, rapid technological innovation, and increasing accessibility, sleep apnea implants are set to play an increasingly vital role in sleep medicine over the next decade.

Regulatory Challenges in Implant Approval

The path from a promising sleep implant concept to an approved medical device available to patients is long and filled with regulatory challenges. These hurdles, while sometimes frustrating for manufacturers and patients awaiting new options, serve a crucial purpose: ensuring that devices are safe, effective, and truly beneficial before they reach the market.

Perhaps the most significant hurdle that manufacturers face is generating sufficient clinical evidence to prove both safety and efficacy. Unlike medications that might be tested on thousands of patients, implantable devices often receive initial approval based on smaller studies—but these must be exceptionally well-designed.

For manufacturers, this creates several challenges:

- Patient recruitment: Finding suitable participants who meet specific criteria
- Long-term follow-up: Tracking outcomes for extended periods (often 1-5 years)

- Comparison standards: Demonstrating superiority or non-inferiority to existing treatments

When Inspire Medical Systems sought approval for its hypoglossal nerve stimulator, its pivotal STAR trial needed to show effectiveness in a specific patient population who had failed CPAP therapy. The trial required multiple sleep lab visits per participant and years of follow-up data—a resource-intensive process that smaller companies often struggle to fund.

Navigating Different Regulatory Frameworks

Sleep apnea affects patients worldwide, but manufacturers must navigate distinct regulatory systems across different countries and regions. This creates a complex patchwork of requirements that can delay the global availability of new treatments.

The three major regulatory frameworks include:

- FDA (United States): Typically requires Premarket Approval (PMA) for implantable devices, the most stringent pathway
- CE Mark (European Union): Often allows earlier market entry but has increasingly stringent requirements under the new Medical Device Regulation (MDR)
- PMDA (Japan): Has unique requirements for clinical evidence, often necessitating studies in Japanese populations

Post-Approval Monitoring and Risk Management

Securing initial approval is just the beginning. Manufacturers face ongoing regulatory requirements for post-market surveillance, adverse event reporting, and quality control. These systems help ensure long-term safety but create substantial operational demands.

For sleep implants, this includes:

- Tracking device performance in real-world settings
- Monitoring and investigating adverse events

Effective post-approval monitoring ensures that any issues are promptly addressed, maintaining patient safety and device reliability over time.

Patient Empowerment and Educational Strategies

Traditional patient education often focused simply on providing instructions—how to use a device, when to schedule follow-ups, and what side effects to watch for. While these basics remain important, modern approaches recognize that truly effective education goes much deeper.

Research backs this up. Studies show that comprehensive patient education programs can improve sleep apnea treatment adherence by 30-40% compared to basic instruction alone. For patients with implantable devices, education has been linked to:

- Higher satisfaction with treatment outcomes
- Better management of device settings and features
- More effective communication with healthcare providers
- Greater improvement in quality of life measures

Effective Educational Strategies

The most successful patient education approaches combine multiple strategies tailored to different learning styles and needs. Here are the approaches showing the strongest results:

Multi-Modal Learning

People absorb information differently—some learn best by reading, others by watching demonstrations, and still others through hands-on practice. Effective education programs incorporate all these approaches:

- Visual aids: Anatomical models, animated videos, and visual guides that show exactly how sleep apnea affects the body and how implants address the problem
- Interactive demonstrations: Hands-on opportunities to handle demo devices and practice using remote controls or other patient-operated components
- Written materials: Clear, jargon-free guides that patients can reference at home, ideally written at an 8th-grade reading level
- Verbal instruction: Face-to-face explanations with opportunities to ask questions

Peer Support Programs

One of the most powerful educational tools is connecting patients with others who have firsthand experience with sleep implants. Peer support programs provide both practical knowledge and emotional reassurance that can be difficult to obtain from healthcare providers alone.

These programs offer a platform for patients to share their experiences, challenges, and successes, fostering a community of understanding and support.

Conclusion

As we conclude our exploration of innovations in sleep apnea treatment, let's look ahead to the transformative developments on the horizon that promise to revolutionize patient care further. While this chapter has focused primarily on implantable devices, exciting developments in medication-based treatments are emerging that may complement or even enhance implant therapy. The most promising development comes from medications originally developed for diabetes and weight management. GLP-1 receptor agonists like tirzepatide have shown remarkable effectiveness in treating sleep apnea in clinical trials—particularly in patients with obesity.

Recent clinical trials suggest this combination approach may be particularly effective. In the SURMOUNT-OSA trial, patients receiving both therapies showed nearly double the improvement compared to either treatment alone. The future of sleep apnea treatment increasingly recognizes that the condition rarely exists in isolation. Research by Basheri and colleagues has highlighted the complex interconnections between sleep apnea and conditions like diabetes, heart disease, and metabolic syndrome.

Tomorrow's sleep apnea management will likely take a more holistic approach, addressing these interconnected conditions simultaneously rather than treating them as separate issues. This integrated approach is particularly relevant for patients with implants, as their overall health status directly affects treatment outcomes. For instance, better management of diabetes may enhance the efficacy of sleep apnea treatments, leading to improved patient care and quality of life.

www.ingramcontent.com/pod-product-compliance
Lightning Source LLC
LaVergne TN
LVHW021238080526
838199LV00088B/4579